THE PPO HANDBOOK

S. Brian Barger
President
Morgan Bigae Institute
Cincinnati, Ohio

David G. Hillman
Vice-President
Morgan Bigae Institute
Cincinnati, Ohio

H. Randall Garland
Executive Vice-President
Health Planning and Resource
Development Association of the
Central Ohio River Valley
Cincinnati, Ohio

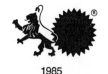

AN ASPEN PUBLICATION®
Aspen Systems Corporation

1985

Rockville, Maryland
Royal Tunbridge Wells

Library of Congress Cataloging in Publication Data

Barger, S. Brian
The PPO handbook.

Includes bibliographies and index.
1. Preferred provider organizations (Medical care)
I. Hillman, David G. II. Garland, H. Randall. III Title. IV. Title: PPO handbook.
RA413.B27   1985   362.1   84-20371
ISBN: 0-89443-569-8

Publisher: John R. Marozsan
Associate Publisher: Jack W. Knowles, Jr.
Editor-in-Chief: Michael B. Brown
Executive Managing Editor: Margot G. Raphael
Managing Editor: M. Eileen Higgins
Editorial Services: Martha Sasser
Printing and Manufacturing: Debbie Collins

Library of Congress Catalog Card Number: 84-20371
ISBN: 0-89443-569-8

Printed in the United States of America

1 2 3 4 5

To our parents,

Curt and Helen,

David and Phyllis,

Howard and Lida.

Our thanks for the

love,

wisdom,

inspiration,

and

sacrifices.

We love you.

Table of Contents

Preface

The decade of the 1980s has produced a wealth of societal changes. The computer explosion, industrial decline, and nuclear proliferation are but a few of the issues profoundly reshaping the way we live and behave. The health care environment, too, is experiencing unparalleled and unprecedented changes.

The preferred provider arrangement today occupies a unique, almost symbolic, position in health care's ambiguous environment. The PPO represents, in microcosm, all of the changes, innovations, uncertainties, and concerns occurring throughout the medical system. Financing innovations, provider survival, the emergence of private-sector review, new-found purchaser aggressiveness, to name but a few, are embedded in the PPO movement.

The phenomenal interest generated by preferred provider programs has resulted in the preparation of numerous materials on the subject. A number of "show and tell" articles have highlighted the basic characteristics, structure, and operating environments of individual PPOs. Select monographs have dissected the plethora of issues, contractual and otherwise, that physicians, hospitals, and purchasers must consider when PPO participation is offered. Other materials have methodically detailed the "how to's" of development and administration.

All of these have served a valuable purpose. At the same time, though, the frenzied pace of PPO activity has produced, and will likely continue to produce, crowded alternative delivery system markets in many communities. And with such crowding has come the need for PPOs to distinctly differentiate themselves from the crowd. This important ability to differentiate, to excel in crowded medical markets, requires more than the standard array of PPO literature. It requires new perspectives, innovative techniques, and creative, pragmatic instruments for the future PPO.

That is the purpose of this book. Physicians, hospitals, and preferred panel arrangements that constantly innovate and pursue new horizons will survive, even thrive, in the medical marketplace of the future. This book has been written for those who aspire to embrace such a destiny.

Throughout this work we have (1) reported on interesting and creative activities of individual preferred provider programs, (2) outlined different perspectives, and (3) attempted to advance the PPO movement by articulating untried but thoughtful suggestions. For example, the reader will find our view of the historical evolution of PPOs and their probable future to be thought provoking if not controversial. The same can be said about our somewhat nontraditional views of antitrust considerations. Technical approaches to the selection of physicians and hospitals, physician payment systems like the Physician Incentive Account (PIA), and financial methods for assessing PPO impact on purchasers and hospitals each offer the reader new tools for grappling with some of the most difficult PPO-related matters. We are convinced that those considering PPO involvement or development, and those already in its midst, will benefit, conceptually and operationally, from that which is new, novel, and futuristic.

S. Brian Barger
David G. Hillman
H. Randall Garland

Part I

The Evolution and Status of Preferred Provider Organizations

Chapter 1

The Evolution of Preferred Provider Organizations

The Physicians' Alliance for Medical Excellence is a nonprofit corporation composed of independent physicians in the Lexington, Kentucky, metropolitan area. Formal participation in the Alliance during 1983 required that physicians pay an annual membership fee of $1,000, present their 1981 Blue Cross utilization profile for examination, submit their practice to ongoing peer review, and limit future fee increases to the rate of increase in the consumer price index. The stiff financial and membership criteria have not inhibited the growth of the young organization, which now has over 120 physicians. Because the Alliance has been able to statistically demonstrate to employers in the area that member physicians are 15 percent less costly than comparable practitioners they expect to save subscribing employers hundreds of thousands of dollars each year—and, in doing so, ensure the future viability and growth of their own practices in an increasingly competitive health care market.

The early 1980s have been a time of many changes for the health care system in the United States. The ways of the past decades have been and continue to be involuntarily discarded. A new set of ground rules is being incrementally planted in their place. This revolution has been given many different labels. It has been called competition; it has been referred to as a price sensitivity. Regardless of its name, the revolution heralds dramatic, new approaches to the delivery of medical care in the United States. At the center of this revolution is the Preferred Provider Organization (PPO). This price-competitive health delivery arrangement, which we will shortly describe and examine in depth, is considered by some to be the panacea for controlling medical care inflation. Others view the PPO as nothing more than a creative marketing scheme devised by aggressive health providers. Irrespective of one's personal perspective, it is abundantly clear that the emergence of preferred provider organizations will not leave the health care system unaltered.

WHY THE PPO EXPLOSION?

By definition, a preferred provider organization is a formal arrangement whereby the services of a select panel of health care providers are marketed on the basis of cost efficiency to purchasers, for which payment is on a prospectively negotiated, predominantly fee-for-service basis, and in which subscribers have an economic incentive to use the select panel. The essence of the PPO is its brokering function (Figure 1-1). Regardless of sponsorship, a preferred provider arrangement behaves like a middleman between (1) the purchasers of health care and (2) the suppliers of medical services—physicians and hospitals. By bringing major purchasers of care together, a PPO measurably increases their buying power, resulting in controlled or reduced health costs. Providers of care participate in this arrangement because they recognize the advantage of having access to potentially large pools of business in an increasingly competitive health care marketplace.

PPO growth in just a few years has been phenomenal. In 1981, it was estimated that less than ten preferred panel arrangements were operational. Current estimates have placed the number of PPOs at well over 100 (see Table 1-1).

But prototypes have existed for several decades.[1] In fact, low-cost medical services were offered to California employee benefit groups by panels of physicians in the late 1800s. Insurance carriers in the states of Washington and Oregon directly and prospectively negotiated inpatient and outpatient rates as early as 1910 for patients requiring care under the then newly enacted workers' compensation laws. In 1939 the California Physicians' Service marketed medical services to purchaser groups, requiring that participating physicians accept the Service's payment as full reimbursement for select categories of patients. The concept of physician contracting was eventually broadened by the evolution of Blue Shield plans across the United States. In a similar fashion, Foundations for Medical Care (FMC), which had their origin in the early 1950s, have used the usual, customary, and reasonable (UCR) fee structure for determining the maximum fee payable to participating physicians when services are rendered to FMC enrollees. At the hospital level, negotiated, discounted payments have been a component of Blue Cross contracts in many states.

PPO-like arrangements in various forms, then, have been present for some time. Why has such unusual and dramatic growth occurred in the last few years? The answer to this question can best be obtained by considering the influence of four interrelated factors. First, serious purchaser concern over escalating medical expenditures gained momentum in the late 1970s and early 1980s as

Figure 1-1 The Preferred Provider Arrangement

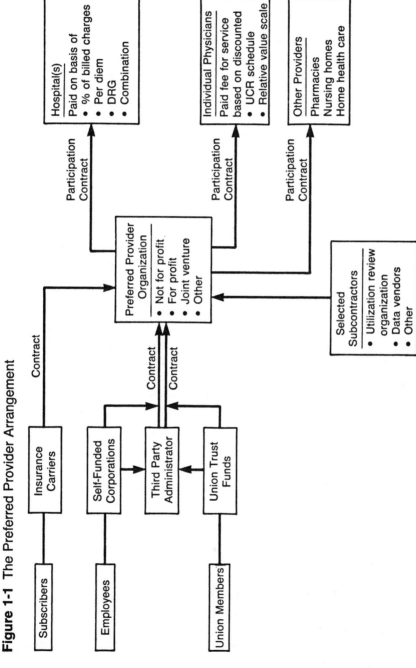

Table 1-1 The Growth of Preferred Provider Organizations, 1982–1984

Date	Number (Developing and/or Operational)	Source
February 1982	6	Interstudy Survey
September 1982	40	American Hospital Association Survey
June 1983	64	American Medical Care and Review Assoc. (*PPO Directory*)
October 1983	107	American Medical Care and Review Assoc. (*PPO Directory*)
January 1984	123	American Medical Care and Review Assoc. (*PPO Directory*)

the result of adverse economic conditions and medical inflation. Second, this pressure forced major purchasers to consider new arrangements to control rapidly escalating medical care expenditures. Third, these same purchasers were afforded the opportunity of observing, in California and in Denver, Colorado, sizable cost-containment gains achieved through provider contracting and negotiation. Last, these and other trends did not go unnoticed by health institutions and physicians. There was a clear acknowledgment on the part of the provider community that future survival would depend on the ability to compete on the basis of price. The surplus of physicians and the erosion of hospital market shares because of HMO growth suggested that financial hardships awaited those who failed to creatively address emerging price sensitivity. Exhibit 1-1 outlines conditions and the economic climate that evolved.

BUSINESS AND INDUSTRY RESPOND TO PRESSURES FOR COST CONTROL

Major purchasers of health care such as large corporations and union trust funds have been disturbed about spiraling health costs for some time. Until the late '70s, however, purchaser attitudes were typically polite, though concerned. The influence of a sluggish economy on corporate profits, competitiveness, and survival, however, changed this situation significantly. As one executive put it bluntly in conversation, "The fact that rising health care costs were the single largest growing expenditure in the corporate budget took on new meaning for those corporations in highly competitive industries, such as the food industry, in which the margin is typically one-half of one percent or less." The economic

Exhibit 1-1 Trends Providing a Receptive Environment for the Rapid Expansion of PPOs

National economic changes force purchaser response:	• Medical inflation was unusually high. • The capital expenditure boom in the early 1980s seemed to offer little hope that costs would moderate on their own. • The economy in general slowed. • Unemployment was high.
Purchaser sought relief from adverse economic conditions:	• Self-funding became attractive. • Employees were presented with greater cost sharing. • Business/purchaser coalitions grew quickly. • Purchasers began comparing health provider cost efficiency. • Competition was viewed as the desired solution to medical inflation.
Purchasers observed approaches to cost containment that produced price sensitivity in the health market:	• California's Medi-Cal initiated select hospital contracting. • Denver's PPO arrangements attracted national attention.
Health providers saw excess resources and new financing arrangements:	• A surplus of physicians was observed. • HMOs were successfully attracting patients. • Private sector utilization review was reducing hospital utilization and occupancy rates. • "Convenience" ambulatory care centers were attracting patients. • DRGs became a reality.

difficulties of the early 1980s, characterized by high unemployment, large federal deficits, and the concomitant lack of investor faith in the industrial sector demanded that corporations aggressively seek out any and all tools for reducing operating costs. Bulging corporate health benefit expenditures were a natural starting point.

Looking back over the last several years, we can see that two generic postures were assumed by major corporate purchasers. Each of these has served to provide fertile ground for the explosion of the PPO movement—and its continuation into the immediate future. The first posture can be described as one of increased employee cost sharing. The economic climate of the early '80s forced labor negotiators to consider, for the first time, the sharing of financial risk between employer and employee.[2] Some of these efforts were successful. Others weren't; several labor disputes erupting in 1983 (AT&T, Greyhound Corporation, Container Corporation of America) resulted from benefit cutback attempts.[3] The trend toward employee cost sharing has been a significant factor influencing PPO development because, quite simply, PPO evolution requires economic incentives or disincentives that encourage consumers to use a select panel of providers.

The second posture assumed by corporate purchasers concerned health insurance. The adverse economy stimulated efforts on the part of the business sector to seek out alternatives to traditional health coverage, the cost of which had (has) been doubling every three to five years. The alternative frequently chosen has been, in retrospect, predictable.

THE ABANDONMENT OF TRADITIONAL INSURANCE

As the cost-containment difficulties of the 1970s expanded into the 1980s, more and more corporations abandoned traditional insurance mechanisms in favor of self-funded or self-insured arrangements (see Table 1-2).

The growth of self-funding has been robust, and with good reason. Among other benefits, self-funding can routinely reduce health benefit costs by 10 percent in the first year of operation and enhance corporate cash flow; cash assets are no longer stored in insurance company reserves. In 1960, approximately 6 percent of all health benefits payments under private insurance programs were made by self-funded groups.[4] Estimates for 1980 ranged from 13 percent to 20 percent.[5] Larger corporations have moved steadily in this direction: 46 percent of Fortune 1000 Corporations were reported as being self-funded in 1982. One health policy expert has predicted that, if current trends continue, self-funding will equal the purchasing power of Blue Cross or that of commercial insurance carriers by 1985.[6]

Table 1-2 The Growth in Self-Funding of Employee Health Benefits

Year	Self-Funded Employee Health Benefit Expenditures as a % of Total Private Health Insurance Payments
1960	6.4%
1970	6.5%
1977	10.7%
1980*	13.2–19%
1985**	33%

*Estimated
**Forecast based on growth

The movement toward self-funding has been an important trend influencing eventual PPO development for two reasons. Companies that have become self-funded have access to a greater level of data and information and have become familiar with both the size and growth of medical care bills. Also, self-funding has increased both the perception and reality of financial risk. In turn, these two factors have seemingly encouraged major corporate purchasers to apply common business principles to the purchase of medical care. A fundamental principle of any well-managed business operation is volume purchasing. If one purchases greater amounts of a product, one typically expects a more favorable price. Health care, in many respects, is being viewed for the first time in a similar light.

BUSINESS/PURCHASER COALITIONS

The unusual and rapid growth of business/purchaser coalitions has also provided a foundation for the evolution of the PPO movement. Before 1980, there were less than 40 coalitions. In 1982 there were 50. Today the number is quickly approaching 150 coalitions (see Table 1-3).

The rapid expansion of purchaser coalitions has been important to the evolution of PPOs because coalitions have provided the community base from which major purchasers could initiate various types of collective cost-containment action and, more specifically, from which support for preferred provider organizations and other cost-efficient systems could originate. Coalitions have undertaken, collectively, many projects that have contributed to the present national interest in PPOs.[7] One has been particularly noteworthy. The collection of institution-specific health cost data has served to identify the substantial differences in the cost and utilization experience of individual hospitals. A natural question resulting from such analyses concerned provider efficiency. The data hinted to business coalitions, and continues to illustrate to them, that large differences exist in the cost-containment and utilization performance of individual providers.[8]

Armed with data indicating, at least on the surface, that major discrepancies exist between the cost performance of individual providers, coalitions and their members have been instrumental in facilitating the evolution of preferred provider

Table 1-3 The Rapid Growth of Business/Purchaser Health Coalitions

Year	Number of Coalitions
1980	20
1981	59
1982	95
1983	105
1984 (Est.)	170

organizations, which, conceptually, are designed to exclude inefficient institutions. At least part of the pro-PPO orientation can be traced to the corporate sector's perspective concerning the manner in which health care costs should be controlled. In general, business and industrial purchasers have supported competitive approaches to cost containment as opposed to regulatory ones.

It is ironic, yet very significant, that one of the procompetitive actions undertaken by the business-supported Republican administration backfired and, in its failure, provided a springboard for increased corporate concern over rising health benefit costs. This was the attempt in 1981 to disband and defund the national health planning program.[9] Between 1981 and 1983, a third of the community-based planning bodies were eliminated, with federal funding for the entire program being reduced by about 60 percent. This interruption, in the admittedly less-than-perfect planning network, offered an opportunity for many institutional providers to undertake new capital investments. They did so, and continue to do so, in an unparalleled manner.

THE CAPITAL EXPENDITURE BOOM: FUELING PURCHASER CONCERNS

The attempt to disband the health planning system paved the way for seemingly unlimited provider capital activity, which, in the end, has greatly fueled purchaser concerns about future levels of health care inflation. Various studies have attempted to estimate the relationship between capital expenditures and additional hospital operating costs. A general rule of thumb has been that $1 of capital investment produces 30¢ to 50¢ of additional operating costs.[10] Studies on the construction of new hospitals have shown even higher operating increases.

Health care purchasers have also been well aware that large amounts of hospital capital investment were (and are) being funded by extremely costly debt instruments. But their greatest concern has not been solely the relationship between capital and operating costs; nor has it been merely the extensive use of debt. Rather, it has been formulated heavily on the observation that the hospital system in the U.S. is undergoing staggering levels of capital investment. Estimates of this capital investment have ranged from $100 billion to $200 billion for the decade of the '80s (see Table 1-4). This is equal to approximately two to three times the investment undertaken during the 1970s.[11] If this trend continues, as it appears it might, some health experts have estimated that 60 percent of all community hospital beds in operation in 1980 will have been renovated or remodeled by the conclusion of this building boom.

Health care purchasers have, with justification, become increasingly alarmed about future rates of medical inflation. Not only have purchasers experienced the traumatic growth (and inflation) of the late '70s and the early '80s; it appears that these may have only been mild harbingers of escalation in the future.

Table 1-4 Certificate of Need Approvals in Selected States, 1980 and 1982

State	Certificate of Need Approvals (Millions of Dollars)	
	1980	*1982*
Ohio	$435	$914
California	202	655
Mississippi	74	150
Georgia	173	302
Texas	560	1,319
New York	369	843
Wyoming	8	71

Source: Abstracted from American Health Planning Association, *Report to AHPA Members* (May 1983).

By the early 1980s, health care purchasers were, out of necessity, becoming militant. They were faced with uncontrollable medical budgets and foresaw serious problems for the future. Corporations were assuming greater levels of risk through the process of self-funding. The changing economy and its influence on the competitiveness of major industries demanded new and novel cost-control approaches. American business and industry were ready for solutions to the cost problems. They were organizing themselves in coalitions. Many were leaning toward competitive models.[12]

At about the same time, two competitive-oriented programs gained national prominence and visibility. The first was a relatively new, Denver-based health delivery system called Mountain Medical Affiliates. The second program was the select hospital contracting effort undertaken by the California Medicaid Program, Medi-Cal. These two programs, because of the high visibility and strong emphasis on the application of common business principles, offered purchasers, at least in concept, a sweeping new approach to cost containment.

THE CALIFORNIA EXPERIMENT: NECESSITY BECOMES THE MOTHER OF INVENTION

The stimulus for the implementation of California's innovative select hospital contracting program can be traced to the passage in 1978 of Proposition 13. This proposition dramatically reduced state taxes and, concomitantly, revenues for state programs, including Medi-Cal.[13]

The Medi-Cal reform proposal (AB 799) was enacted in June 1982. Its focal point was the establishment of the Governor's Office Special Hospital Negotiator (GOSHN). The objective was for the office to enter into individual contracts with "cost efficient" hospitals for the provision of care to Medi-Cal partici-pants.[14] Nongovernmental buyers of health care, particularly insurance com-panies, became highly disturbed by the Medi-Cal changes, fearing that savings reaped by the state would resurface as costs shifted by hospitals to insurance carriers. To make matters worse, existing state law prohibited insurance carriers from obtaining alternative (discounted and otherwise) payment rates from hos-pitals. The insurance industry in the state proposed a companion piece of leg-islation allowing the establishment of and participation in select contracting programs.

The law became effective July 1, 1983; it was both preceded and followed by what can only be described as PPO-mania. Though the Medi-Cal program has been controversial and not without litigation, its impact on cost control has been substantial. Initial estimates suggested that the program would save ap-proximately $200 million in its first year of operation. The eyes and ears of the purchaser sector turned sharply to the West.

COLORADO AND THE PPO MOVEMENT:
UNIQUE CIRCUMSTANCES AND COMMON SENSE

A unique set of circumstances in Denver, Colorado, produced a highly re-ceptive environment for the evolution of preferred provider organizations in the late 1970s and early 1980s. A mobile, growing population, excess health re-sources in the community, and an unusual level of self-funding merged to provide this favorable environment.

Perhaps one of the most significant aspects of the Denver situation was its health benefits arrangements. One benefits consulting organization provided con-sulting and advisory services to groups accounting for almost 400,000 persons in the area. Further, roughly 40 percent of the major corporations in the area were self-funded. By the late 1970s, it was only natural that the benefits con-sulting company would apply business-oriented purchasing practices to Denver's health marketplace. On behalf of its sizable client base, the company began to negotiate volume purchasing arrangements with several hospitals in the Denver metropolitan area. The initial interaction provided a rapid breeding ground for the eventual development of several preferred provider organizations in Denver, most notably Mountain Medical Affiliates, Inc.[15]

PHYSICIANS AND HOSPITALS READ THE HANDWRITING
ON THE WALL

Health providers did not ignore the novel programs in California and Colorado; and they paid constant attention to the growing aggressiveness of the purchaser, particularly corporate, sector.[16] Existing anxieties were only heightened by the advance of new payment systems (reimbursement based on Diagnosis Related Groups—DRGs) and noticeable changes in the flow and magnitude of patient markets brought on by convenient medical clinics, ambulatory surgical facilities, and generally greater competition among health providers. Indeed, this was the poignant message of the early 1980s for providers: fewer patients, fewer dollars, and more providers mean fewer dollars to those who lose the patients.

The growing surplus of physicians and the surprising expansion of health maintenance organizations are two factors commonly associated with PPO emergence.

In 1980 the Graduate Medical Education National Advisory Committee (GMENAC) released a series of reports for the Secretary of Health and Human Services identifying the magnitude of the imminent physician surplus. Projections estimated that an overall physician surplus would approximate 70,000 physicians by the year 1990 and would double by the year 2000 to a level of almost 145,000 physicians (see Table 1-5).[17]

Health maintenance organizations have had a similar competitive impact on the medical community. In 1970, there were 41 health maintenance organizations. By 1982 the number had steadily increased to 265 HMOs. Projections by the U.S. Government's Office of Health Maintenance Organizations suggest that there will be 440 HMOs by 1988, which may include over 19 million enrollees. The Congressional Budget Office has estimated that actual enrollment may be closer to 50 million enrollees, if certain positive conditions materialize (see Table 1-6).[18]

There is no doubt that the physician surplus and the growth of health maintenance organizations have profoundly affected the way physicians and hospitals view their involvement in preferred provider organizations. In almost every community in which PPOs have grown quickly, they have done so because of concern by physicians and hospitals about these two trends. The prospect of dwindling market shares or patient volume and the concurrent introduction of

---

Table 1-5 Aggregate Physician Supply and Requirements, 1978 and Estimates for 1990 and 2000

	Year		
	1978	*1990*	*2000*
Physician Supply	374,800	535,750	642,950
Physician Requirements	418,550	466,000	498,250
Surplus (Shortage)	(43,750)	69,750	144,200

Source: *Report of the Graduate Medical Education National Advisory Committee to the Secretary, Department of Health and Human Services*, vol. II (Washington, D.C.: U.S. Department of Health and Human Services, 1980) PHS-HRA.

Table 1-6 The Growth of Health Maintenance Organizations

Year	Number of HMOs	Estimated Enrollment
1970	41	2.9 million
1974	183	5.3 million
1979	229	8.8 million
1982*	265	10.5 million
1988	442	19.1 million
1989	Not Reported	17.8–46.5 million

*As reported in *Group Health News* (March 1983): 3.

Source: Office of Health Maintenance Organizations, *Prospectus on Health Maintenance Organizations* (Rockville, Md.: Department of Health and Human Services, October 1981), 2, 7.

new financing mechanisms such as DRG-based payment and statewide programs like Medi-Cal and Arizona's AHCCCS (Arizona Health Care Cost Containment System) have made the potential impact of this competition a powerful incentive for provider PPO participation or development.

THE MESSAGE OF THE FUTURE: COMPETITION AND PRICE SENSITIVITY

The half decade preceding 1984 gave birth to a unique culmination of certain societal and health-related changes that have inalterably affected the future of the medical care system in the U.S. The unusual, tumultuous environment of this future will be characterized by increasing levels of price sensitivity and true economic competition between physicians, hospitals, and other providers. The sellers' market of the past, in which payment levels and methods were seemingly dictated, is giving way to the buyers' market of tomorrow. And in this market the purchasers will set the ground rules of price and payment.

There will be winners and there will be losers. Physicians and other medical providers seriously acknowledging the presence of competition and price sensitivity will see this as a time of opportunity and gain. Health providers who have the ability and the vision to creatively organize themselves in efficient, competitive ways will survive and, indeed, thrive during the years to come.

NOTES

1. Joan B. Trauner, *Preferred Provider Organizations: The California Experiment* (San Francisco: University of California, August 1983), 8–9; Boyd Thompson, "AAFMC Report," *UFMC Newsletter 2*, no. 4 (Winter 1982–83): 1.

2. Lorrie Gibson, "Many Employers Hike Deductibles, Premiums," *Business Insurance* (March 12, 1984): 16–17; "Salaried Workers Share Health Costs with Ford," *Business Insurance* (August

15, 1983): 4; Steve Taravella, "High-Tech Firms Redesigning High Cost Plans," *Business Insurance* (March 12, 1984): 1+.

3. "AT&T Strike," *Business Insurance* (August 15, 1984): 4; A. Andry, "210 Strike Over Proposal to Shift Health Care Costs," *Cincinnati Post* (August 29, 1983).

4. M.S. Carroll and R.H. Arnett III, "Private Health Insurance Plans in 1977: Coverage Enrollment and Financial Experience," *Health Care Financing Review* (Fall 1979): 3–22.

5. Greater St. Louis Health Systems Agency, *Health Cost Management: A Review of Major Strategies* (St. Louis: The Greater St. Louis Health Systems Agency, March 1982), 2.

6. J.C. Goldsmith, "Capital Planning Strategies in an Era of Changing Ground Rules," *Trustee* (January 1983): 32.

7. Christine Olson, Business Labor and Health Series No. 1: *Purchaser Health Care Cost Containment Initiatives* (San Francisco: Western Center for Health Planning, October 1981), 1–30.

8. Gerald A. Gleeson, "Case Studies in Private Sector Initiatives: Utilization Review," in *The Dimensions of Health Care Reimbursement* (Madison, Wisc.: The Institute for Health Planning, June 1983), 103–116; The Clearinghouse on Business Coalitions For Health Action, "The Philadelphia (Health) Story: Oldest Coalition Reports Newest Results," *Coalition Report* 3, no. 6 (June 1984): 1.

9. Linda E. Demkovich, "Hospitals' Building and Buying Binge Tied to Cuts in Federal Planning Aid," *National Journal* 17 (April 23, 1983): 832–836.

10. S. Brian Barger and David G. Hillman, *Controlling Medical Costs During the 1980s: A Bold Challenge to The Cincinnati Corporate Community* (Cincinnati: The Greater Cincinnati Chamber of Commerce, July 1983), 16.

11. Alpha Center, *Setting Affordable Units on Capital Expenditures* (Bethesda: Alpha Center, November–December 1982), 1; C. Bradford, G. Caldwell, and J. Goldsmith, "The Hospital Capital Crisis: Issues for Trustees," *Harvard Business Review* (September–October 1982): 56–68.

12. Alison Kittrell, "Firms Promote Health Care Competition: Study," *Business Insurance* (May 28, 1984): 42–43.

13. B.A. Myers, "Public Sector Reimbursement Reform: California's Medi-Cal," in *The Dimensions of Health Care Reimbursement* (Madison, Wisc: The Institute for Health Planning, June 1983), 43–58.

14. "Competition: California Takes the Lead," *Washington Report on Medicine and Health—Perspectives* (September 6, 1982): 1–4.

15. G. Brukart, "Mountain Medical PPO: A Case History of Marketing a New Concept in the Denver Area," *FAH Review* (July/August 1982): 29–32; L.K. Ellwin and D.D. Gregg, *An Introduction to Preferred Provider Organizations* (Excelsion, Minn.: Interstudy, April 1982), Appendix D.

16. Robert Cassidy, "Will the PPO Movement Freeze You Out?" *Medical Economics* (April 18, 1983): 262–274; Harry Schwartz, "California Medicine: Foreshadowing The Future," *Private Practice* (June 1983): 41–45; Esther Fritz Kuntz, "Hospitals Forming PPOs to Fend Off HMO Rivals," *Modern Health Care* 13, no. 2 (February 1983): 22–24.

17. Modeling, Research and Data Technical Panel, *Report to the Graduate Medical Education National Advisory Committee to the Secretary, Department of Health and Human Services*, vol. II (Washington, D.C.: U.S. Department of Health and Human Services, 1980), 273.

18. Office of Health Maintenance Organizations, *Prospectus on Health Maintenance Organizations* (Rockville, Md.: Department of Health and Human Services, October 1981), 7.

Chapter 2

Preferred Provider Organizations: Definition and Characteristics

Regardless of how individual providers, consumers, or purchasers feel about PPOs, a set of certain characteristics is shared by most groups that call themselves preferred provider organizations.

A preferred provider organization may be defined as a formal arrangement whereby the services of a select panel of health care providers are marketed on the basis of cost efficiency to purchasers, for which payment is on a prospectively negotiated, predominantly fee-for-service basis, and in which subscribers have an economic incentive to use the select panel.

There will always be some inconsistency with any definition that is offered for any entity. The same is true for PPOs. There are some organizations that do not prospectively negotiate hospital or physician rates; they feel it is not necessary because they include a highly efficient group of physicians. Also, not all payment to preferred provider organizations is based on the fee-for-service model. Though a majority of payment to PPO physicians is fee-for-service based, there are some groups that have employed a capitation payment arrangement. Economic incentives for consumers also vary greatly; select preferred provider organizations may offer an economic incentive to use the PPO, while others provide a disincentive if the preferred panel is not used.

Even though variations occur, the above definition provides a reasonable generic framework from which to explore the status and operations of this novel alternative medical services delivery system. Exhibit 2-1 presents examples of the many different arrangements.

We should also point out that the term ''preferred provider organization'' is grossly and uniquely inexact.[1] PPOs may be neither preferred nor organizations. Rarely can the providers be considered preferred by purchasers since they are usually not prospectively identified by either purchasers or consumers. Most frequently, providers must meet a series of criteria devised by the PPO, the purpose of which is to differentiate the efficient and capable from the inefficient

Exhibit 2-1 A Summary Compendium of PPO Variations

Scope	Examples
Hospital employees only	Good Samaritan Hospital, Cincinnati, Ohio
Statewide	Ohio Health Choice, Cleveland Ohio
Multi-state/national	Voluntary Hospitals of America, Texas
Sponsorship	
Physician/hospital joint venture	Preferred Health Care, Colorado Springs, Colorado (Associated with Penrose Community Hospitals)
Physician	United PPO, Inc. (sponsored by the United Foundation for Medical Care), San Francisco, California
Hospital network	Mid-America Health Network, Kansas City, Missouri
Multihospital system	Lutheran Hospital Society of Southern California (Universal Health Network)
Third party administrator	AdMar Corporation (Med Network) Santa Ana, California
Insurance carrier	Blue Cross of California (Prudent Buyer Plan), Oakland, California
Government	State of California (Medi-Cal), Sacramento, California
Employer	Edison Company of Southern California, Los Angeles, California
Labor union	Michigan Conference of Teamsters Welfare Fund, Michigan
HMO	AV MED PPO Miami, Florida
Community-based	San Diego Program for Affordable Health Care
Structure	
Not for profit	Princeton PPO (associated with Baptist Medical Center—Princeton), Birmingham, Alabama
For profit	ScrippsCare (associated with Scripps Memorial Hospital), San Diego, California
Physician Selection	
Staff members only	Preferred Health Professionals (Baptist Medical Center) Kansas City, Missouri
Physician invited only after review of practice efficiency data	Greater Baltimore Preferred Provider Organization, Baltimore, Maryland
Physicians selected by physician peers (initially)	Independence Medical Systems, Clearwater, Florida
Participation criteria requires release of practice pattern information	Physicians' Alliance, Lexington, Kentucky (Data from Blue Cross)
	Mid-America Health Network, Kansas City, Missouri (Data from utilization review organization)

Exhibit 2-1 continued

Payment Mechanisms	*Examples*
Discount from UCR, fee for service	Consumer Med, Cincinnati, Ohio
Discount using relative value scale, fee for service	Princeton Preferred Provider Organization, Birmingham, Alabama
UCR or no discount, fee for service	Choice (Aetna Insurance Company), Chicago, Illinois
Capitation (primary care providers) and fee for service (specialists)	Cubic/Scripps Plan (associated with Cubic Corporation and Scripps Clinic), San Diego, California
Hospital: Billed charges with no discount	Preferred Health Professionals, Kansas City, Missouri
Hospital: Billed charges with discount	CompMed (associated with St. John Medical Center), Tulsa, Oklahoma
Hospital: Per diem	San Diego Preferred Provider Organization (associated with the San Diego Foundation for Medical Care), San Diego, California
Hospital: DRG or diagnosis-based	TRUST Program (Blue Cross/Blue Shield of Michigan)
Utilization Review	
None required	Greater Baltimore PPO, Baltimore, Maryland
Mandatory preadmission certification, concurrent length of stay and retrospective review	AV MED PPO, Miami, Florida
Non Acute Profile	KeyCare (Blue Cross/Blue Shield of Virginia)

and less capable. Accordingly, they are admitted providers or selected providers. Second, PPOs are arrangements of independent practitioners, facilities, or group practices bound loosely together by formal agreements and contracts. They are decidedly not organizations in the corporate tradition. These remarks are of little more than intellectual interest at this point in PPO evolutionary history. The term has been accepted by participants in the medical care system in the U.S. and common perceptions exist about the nature and shape of these entities. It is with that in mind that this book perpetuates the term.

PRINCIPAL CHARACTERISTICS OF PREFERRED PROVIDER ORGANIZATIONS

With the above considerations in mind, the principal characteristics of the PPO delivery system can be summarized. In general, they are

1. Formal contractual arrangements
2. A select panel of providers

3. An emphasis on cost efficiency
4. Marketing programs directed at purchasers as opposed to consumers
5. Prospective negotiation of payment
6. Economic incentives to encourage selection of the provider panel.

Formal Arrangements

Legal agreements and contracts represent the force that binds preferred provider organizations together. Perhaps no other health care delivery system is so heavily organized around contracts. In the contractual environment, a preferred provider organization, as a legal entity, initiates contracts with several groups. Purchasers of health care may enter into legal agreements to purchase care. Providers of health care, including pharmacies, nursing homes, home health providers, in addition to the system of hospitals and physicians, may also enter into agreements with the PPO entity to provide services to enrollees.

A Select Panel of Health Providers

The center of any PPO is its panel of providers. Conceptually, the panel of providers may be open to any physician, hospital, or other provider. Practically, however, open panel PPOs are nearly impossible. The ineffectiveness of controls would inevitably produce serious financial and marketing problems. On the other hand, a rigid system that permits the arbitrary exclusion of physicians from participation may open the door to antitrust and other legal problems. The establishment of stringent, but fair, criteria suffers further from the problem of quantifying the efficiency and quality of care delivered by physicians desiring PPO affiliation.

The difficulties involved in selecting high-quality, cost-efficient providers have not precluded all groups from establishing screening mechanisms. The Greater Baltimore Preferred Provider Organization, for example, invites physician participation only after certain data on the quantitative cost efficiency of a potential participant's practice has been studied. Both the Mid-America Health Network (Kansas City, Missouri), through its associated physician group (Mid-America Medical Affiliates), and the Physician's Alliance for Medical Excellence (Lexington, Kentucky) stipulate that prospective physician participants must provide written waivers allowing the PPO to assess previous practice efficiency.

Cost Efficiency

Only a handful of PPOs have specified mechanisms or criteria for screening out the highly efficient from the inefficient. Therefore, it has been incumbent upon preferred provider organizations to establish other approaches to ensuring cost efficiency.

In a very real sense, the cost efficiency of individual PPOs will determine their survival in both the short run and the long run. It is cost efficiency that the PPO entity is actually marketing to the health care purchaser sector, one of whose primary interests is cost containment. The PPO, then, will either meet the expectations of this sector and survive or, conversely, fail to meet these needs and fall by the wayside.

There are several ways in which cost efficiency can be approached. The first and most obvious is the selection of cost-efficient physicians and hospitals. Other avenues to cost efficiency include (1) discounts, (2) the establishment of unique payment systems that place the provider at risk for the cost of care, and (3) a wide assortment of control mechanisms, which may include the following: aggressive utilization review, data feedback systems that furnish providers with an understanding of their costly behavior, and incentive systems for physicians.

Discounts

Discounting is one of the concepts most commonly associated with preferred provider organizations. PPOs such as Mountain Medical Affiliates in Denver, Colorado, employ a relative value scale (RVS) in which physicians are paid 80 to 85 percent of the area's UCR (usual, customary, and reasonable) fee. The Princeton Preferred Provider Organization, a program associated with Baptist Medical Center in Birmingham, Alabama, employs an RVS for paying physicians at a rate equivalent to a discounted fee-for-service payment. Other preferred provider organizations like Tulsa's CompMed and Cincinnati's Consumer Med compensate medical practitioners at a predefined level of the UCR fee for the local area. When employing the UCR-based method, the PPO usually qualifies payment by stating that compensation will be at a certain percentile of the UCR. Some preferred provider organizations pay physicians at the 90th percentile, while others pay at the 50th.

Cost efficiency may also result from discounts negotiated with participating hospitals. Typical payment mechanisms for hospitals might include a negotiated reduction from billed charges for each patient. Negotiated reductions are generally many times smaller than that acquired from physicians. Hospital discounts are frequently in the range of 7 to 10 percent. Geographical areas in which low occupancies and excess beds have produced greater competition may be more accepting of larger discounts. San Diego is one such community. One large preferred provider organization there, the San Diego PPO (a component of the San Diego Foundation for Medical Care), has negotiated several discounts in the range of 30 percent. It is reported that one discount (for an unusually high-cost facility) is approximately $600 per day.

Unique Payment Arrangements

Preferred provider organizations are pursuing other types of hospital payment arrangements that include incentives for cost-efficient behavior at inpatient facilities. Two such payment mechanisms are the daily per diem and the per case payment. The per diem provides an all-inclusive payment for each day of hospital care; per case payment provides an all-inclusive payment for individual diagnostic conditions and procedures, irrespective of the length of stay and resources consumed by the patient. These payment mechanisms, however, increase provider financial risk. That is, if an inpatient facility or its associated medical staff confine patients for excessively long periods of time or employ an excessive amount of costly services, the hospital becomes financially liable for those expenses exceeding the negotiated per day or per case payment. On the other hand, an institution may willingly pursue such payment if it has a long history of efficiency. Such institutions see the alternative payment methods not only as an opportunity to recoup costs associated with the provision of care, but also as a mechanism to generate additional profit because of their efficient behavior.

Controls

The selection of cost-efficient providers, the establishment of discounts, and the initiation of new payment mechanisms each, in its own right, contributes to the cost-efficient character of a preferred provider arrangement. Perhaps the most visible and potentially effective are those efforts designed to control or shape physician behavior in a cost-conscious way. Presently, the primary cost control mechanism employed by preferred provider organizations is utilization review. Utilization review (UR) can take several shapes. Preadmission certification, concurrent length of stay review, retrospective claims and appropriateness of care analysis, mandatory second opinions for elective surgery, and utilization review of ambulatory practice patterns represent the major types of UR conducted by preferred provider arrangements. The San Diego PPO, Inc., is an example of a preferred provider organization that has implemented a majority of these concepts.

Even though these represent the primary utilization review tools, other entities employ, or plan to use, different approaches. In Baltimore, for example, the Greater Baltimore PPO does not intend to require any type of utilization review. This is due to the highly selective process used by that organization in the choice of its physicians. At the other end of the continuum is Preferred Health Professionals, located in Kansas City, Missouri. This organization has tailored its program to incorporate only those utilization review procedures requested by particular purchasers. For some purchasers, the utilization controls are intensive and restrictive; for others, only minimal utilization control programs are initiated.

Physician cost efficiency can also be controlled through the use of incentives. Financial incentive models have been employed in prepaid group practices and associated health maintenance organizations. As yet, they have not found an adequate niche within the preferred provider organization movement. One community-based preferred provider organization, the San Diego Program for Affordable Health Care, intends to give serious consideration to the development of physician incentives as that program evolves.[2] The Program is one of a handful of national demonstration projects funded by the Robert Wood Johnson Foundation. The Foundation hopes that this small number of adequately funded projects will provide a unique base of information about effective, results-oriented, cost-containment programs that can be implemented at the community level throughout the United States.

Blue Cross and Blue Shield of Virginia's PPO, KeyCare, has been designed to include specific financial incentives for physicians. The Professional Provider Incentive Program reflects the ability of individual practitioners to reduce hospital admissions and patient days while shifting the provision of care from the inpatient to the outpatient setting. Incentive payments are expected to be made annually.

Physician behavior may also be changed through the use of data feedback systems. Again, data feedback has not been used extensively in preferred provider organizations, with the exception of concurrent utilization review. As noted above, the concurrent length of stay review process identifies the expected patient length of stay for a physician at the time of admission. CompMed, a Tulsa, Oklahoma-based preferred provider organization, has extended this process one step further. Physicians are provided with a cumulative statement of patient charges placed daily on a patient's medical chart. Empirical information on the effectiveness of this approach is not available, although the sponsors of the program believe the data feedback system has influenced physician behavior in a positive, cost-effective way.

Marketing to Health Care Purchasers

Major health care purchasers are clearly the focus of marketing activity. They are also the group that is primarily interested in preferred provider organizations because of the potential for cost containment. For a variety of reasons, early PPOs frequently directed their marketing efforts at self-funded corporations and labor union trusts. The perception was that these groups had a keen interest in PPO participation and, in addition, appeared to be able to incorporate PPOs into benefits packages with a minimum of administrative problems because of their self-funded status. Preferred provider organizations that have developed since 1983 have placed a greater emphasis on attracting all purchasers, including third party administrators, employee benefits brokers, and insurance companies. The perspective here seems to be that a preferred provider organization can better compete with other PPOs to the extent that it covers a larger share of the market. Moreover, marketing only to self-funded organizations limits the expansion potential of any particular PPO's market share.

Negotiated Payment for Health Services

Prospectively negotiated payment for physician, hospital, and other health-related services is the fifth characteristic of a preferred provider organization. Different payment arrangements have been discussed above in generic fashion. Fee-for-service is the most common mode of payment for physician services, while billed charges (and a discount from them) is, at present, the typical mode of payment for hospital services. Rapid payment of bills is an almost universal feature.

Regardless of the type of payment employed, the PPO acts as a broker, prospectively negotiating the level and scope of payment to hospitals, physicians, and other providers.

Economic Incentives for Consumers

Consumers must be motivated to limit their selection of health providers to those participating in the preferred panel. There is little reason for a consumer to select services from a limited group of hospitals and physicians (the PPO) when the universe of hospitals and physicians in the consumer's community is usually available to them through the provisions of traditional health insurance. As a result, PPOs uniformly require that participating purchasers offer their members economic rewards to use the preferred provider organization. Three options are generally employed. The first provides a financial incentive to the employee to use the preferred panel. For example, if an employee's health coverage normally pays 80 percent of the cost of medical services, this coverage might be increased to 100 percent when preferred professionals and facilities are used.

The second type of approach is the use of disincentives. Again, an employee's health coverage may pay for 80 percent of services provided to that individual. Under the disincentive approach, the patient receives this level of coverage only when the preferred panel is used; if it is not used, the coverage may drop to 50 percent. Some researchers believe this latter disincentive-oriented approach is more effective in shaping consumer behavior.

Under the third option, a broader range of services may be available at no cost or limited cost when the preferred panel is used.

THE FOUNDATION OF THE PREFERRED PROVIDER ARRANGEMENT: BENEFITS FOR ALL PARTICIPANTS

In an ideal situation, a preferred provider organization produces economic benefits for each of the three major participants: purchaser, patient, and provider. It is this feature of across-the-board benefits to participants that makes the PPO movement potentially very powerful. Benefits that may accrue to each participant are outlined in Exhibit 2-2.

Purchaser Benefits

Health care purchasers desire one primary result from their involvement with preferred provider arrangements. That is control over medical expenditures. All other benefits that purchasers may derive are born of and secondary to an interest in health care cost containment.

Major health purchasers with knowledge of PPO capabilities are fully aware that up-front discounts represent only temporary, minimal cost savings and control. In situations where existing health services may be priced substantially

---

Exhibit 2-2 Benefits to PPO Participants

Participant	*Benefits*
Purchaser	• Control of medical expenditures through utilization review
	• Savings through negotiated fee arrangement/schedule
	• Decreased financial risk, when incentive-based payment arrangements (per diem, per case) are negotiated
	• Improved protection from cost shifting
	• Ease of administration (in most cases)
Patient	• Choice of geographically dispersed providers
	• First-dollar coverage (frequently) when preferred panel is used
	• Improved quality of care through initiation of utilization/quality review mechanisms
Providers	• Maintenance of traditional forms of payment (fee-for-service)
	• Protection of existing market share
	• Potential expansion of market share
	• Enhancement of cash flow through rapid claims payment
	• Improvement in payment mix of patients
	• Alteration of patient mix

above community averages, the acquired negotiated discounts may not even represent true savings. It is for this reason that purchasers recognize the importance of control mechanisms, specifically utilization review. Benefit costs are controlled in a manner closely paralleling the ability to control hospital utilization. Preliminary information on the ability of preferred arrangements to meet cost containment needs of the purchaser sector are encouraging. Tulsa's CompMed has produced internal data that indicate PPO patients experience hospital costs that are 8 percent less than those of comparable groups. The Physicians' Alliance has quantified employee benefits savings at about 15 percent.[3] Rohr Industries in Chula Vista, California, estimates eventual savings at a similar level.[4] A California-based insurance carrier linked to a third party administrator-sponsored PPO estimated 1981 savings for PPO users to be over 20 percent.[5]

Purchasers also derive other benefits from participation. The use of innovative payment mechanisms, like per diem and DRG-based payment, provides purchasers with the added benefit of risk sharing. Self-funded or self-insured purchasers assume full financial risk for the provision of care to enrollees. When innovative financial mechanisms such as those mentioned above are employed, purchasers share risk with providers. This concept has been appealing to purchasers because it forces greater provider cost consciousness and, ultimately, directly contributes to the overall goal of controlling medical expenditures.

The alteration of employee or union member benefit programs such as the offering of health maintenance organizations, or the initiation of flexible benefits, can produce administrative difficulties for self-funded corporations and labor union trust funds. The preferred provider organization option avoids such pitfalls in that it can, in most cases, be easily integrated into the existing benefits structure of corporations and other purchasers. It is this ease of administration that serves both as an attractive aspect of the PPO and as a benefit for the purchaser.

Employee benefits consultants, brokers, and third party administrators are not technically purchasers, yet each derives certain benefits from participation in preferred arrangements. Major purchasers look to brokers, consultants, and third party administrators for direct and advisory assistance in cost containment. It is in the economic interest of and a competitive advantage for these organizations to be linked with preferred provider organizations. Brokers, consultants, and third party administrators unable to extend innovative cost-containment options to their clients ultimately lose clients to more creative competitors. Accordingly, these groups receive the benefit of maintaining their own market share or increasing it, by actively promoting PPOs.

An example of the impact this involvement can have is typified by the benefits consulting group Martin E. Segal and Company. The Segal organization served as a primary initiator of PPO activity in Denver, Colorado. It has not only increased its general benefits consulting activity as a result of PPO involvement but also initiated a new product: PPO developmental assistance.

Benefits Derived by Consumers

The consumer/patient also derives economic benefits from PPO participation. As we have seen, an economic incentive approach frequently used is the elimination of copayments and deductibles, i.e., 100 percent payment for services rendered. This is in contrast to a typical situation in which the patient is liable for both copayment and the deductible. Also, a consumer not using the preferred panel pays 20 percent of the cost of rendered services. In a disincentive-oriented arrangement, the consumer may have only 50 percent of non-PPO services covered.

In many cases the consumer/patient also benefits from a relatively wide geographic distribution of physicians and hospitals, although this will depend on the particular characteristics of the individual preferred arrangement. It can be expected that, in general, the breadth of patient choice, and the geographical distribution of providers, is greater in preferred provider organizations than in group practice or staff model health maintenance organizations.

Potential for improvements in the quality of care exists. Aggressive utilization control programs are commonplace in preferred provider organizations and these, in combination with their systems and individual physician monitoring, provide an excellent opportunity for closely surveying patient care.

This is not to suggest that all providers agree with this view. There has been a tendency on the part of certain health provider groups to question the quality of care offered. This concern arises from the acknowledgment that PPOs limit choice (because they allow participation only from some subset of all practitioners in a community) and that restrictive utilization controls may affect quality of care. The issue of choice has been one of ongoing and spirited discussion.

Philosophically, choice is always limited. Individuals residing in rural communities many times lack physicians; when physicians are available in rural areas, choice is necessarily limited only to those physicians within reasonable travel time. Choice is also limited for patients of a particular payment status, specifically Medicaid patients. Not all physicians participate in Medicaid programs. As a result, persons receiving Medicaid benefits are required to locate those physicians willing and able to provide care under Medicaid payment arrangements. Again, choice is limited. The same holds true for Medicare participants, inner-city residents, populations using IPAs (Independent Practice Associations) and HMOs. Arguments suggesting that PPOs limit choice any more so than other arrangements are, simply, at variance with the reality of medical care.

Benefits for Providers

Hospitals and physicians, as well as other participating providers, receive numerous benefits from PPO affiliation. The most obvious is the maintenance of existing market shares and patient volumes. Associated with this is the possibility of expanding both market share and volume. A study conducted by the California Hospital Association in the spring of 1983 concluded that 95 percent of hospitals currently contracting with PPOs or in the process of developing PPOs did so in an effort to increase market share; 88 percent were interested in increasing occupancy rates, while 54 percent were pursuing PPO involvement as a general response to marketplace demands.[6]

The rapid claims payment feature of the PPO movement represents a third benefit experienced by health care providers. A consulting firm involved with PPO development has suggested that payments to physicians may frequently take 40 days or more and that 5 percent to 10 percent of accounts may represent collection problems. Hospital collectables can easily be 60 days or more. Payment from PPOs to providers is usually accomplished in seven to ten days, with most PPOs guaranteeing payment within a maximum period (14 days, 30 days). The promptness with which providers are paid typically improves cash flow and, because of the elimination of extensive delays in payment experienced by some providers, increases investment opportunities and, ultimately, revenue.

PPO participation allows hospitals to alter both the mix of patients and the mix of payors in ways beneficial to a facility. For example, an institution experiencing serious occupancy problems with its pediatrics and obstetrics programs, or an organization wishing to initiate such services, may view PPO participation as a meaningful opportunity. The youthful nature of most employee groups, and the mini baby boom occurring in the 1980s, indicate that PPO involvement can facilitate desired patient mix changes. Payment mix alteration, too, can be an important objective. Increases in hospital revenue from greater numbers of full-paying (or almost full-paying) patients is a welcome change from losses at the hands of influencial payors, like Medicare, who may be reimbursing a hospital at levels far below the actual cost of services. Changes in payor mix, such as a reduction in the percent of total revenue derived from Medicare, combined with a simultaneous increase in revenues derived from PPO payment can have a very positive outcome on an institution's bottom line revenue and net operating margin.

Two longer-term advantages must also be mentioned as benefits perceived by health providers. First, the PPO concept, in general, maintains existing forms of health care reimbursement. That is, the majority of physician payment, at least at this time, is fee for service. For hospitals, most payment is designed around billed charges. Both of these payment mechanisms limit provider risk and, further, help ensure that providers are adequately reimbursed for the costs of care.

Second, an unusual, but nonetheless important, benefit to providers is that PPO involvement forces extensive cooperation between hospitals and their medical staffs. This has frequently been absent in the past. The PPO serves, then, as a vehicle for nurturing important working relationships between medical staffs and their hospitals. This not only assists provider involvement in a PPO; it also is an important springboard for future joint hospital/physician activities crucial to the survival of hospitals in an environment of increasing price sensitivity.

NOTES

1. J.R. Kimmey, "A.K.A. PPO: A Review of Selected Provider Arrangements," (Madison, Wisc.: Institute for Health Planning, November 1983), 2–3.

2. For additional information on this program see *Health Care Monitor* (San Diego: The San Diego Employers Health Cost Coalition, 1983); M. LeRoux, "Grants Help Communities Attack Health Costs," *Business Insurance* (March 12, 1984): 36–38.

3. Physicians' Alliance For Medical Excellence, *Policy Statement* (Lexington, Ky.: 1983).

4. Personal communication with executives at Rohr Industries, Chula Vista, California, June 1983.

5. Suzanne Viau, *PPOs: The State of the Art* (Washington, D.C.: Health Publishing Ventures, 1983), 31–32.

6. Perspectives, "Preferred Providers Proliferate," *Washington Report on Medicine and Health* (June 20, 1983): 3.

Chapter 3

The Distribution, Dimensions, and Impact of PPOs

Charting the evolution of preferred provider arrangements is made difficult by their rapid growth. Equally as difficult is accurately tracing PPO distribution, form, and relationship to other service delivery and insurance-like programs. In this chapter, we have chosen to illuminate these matters in cross-section, rather than make a sprawling and likely futile attempt to cover them for all time.

WHERE AND WHY HAVE PPOs DEVELOPED?

As of late 1983, official estimates reported more than 120 PPOs either in existence or in developmental stages in the United States. A two-thirds majority were in an operational phase; the remainder were preoperational. Twenty-nine states and the District of Columbia reported preferred provider organization activity. California led the list with 49 PPOs, followed by Ohio, Florida, and Colorado, each with 7.[1] Professionals involved with PPO development unofficially estimated the number of PPOs to be around 400 at the beginning of 1984 with as many as 150 of these in California.

Table 3-1 shows that over 50 statistical metropolitan areas (formerly standard metropolitan statistical areas) recorded operational or preoperational PPO activity in the winter of 1984. The favorable legislative climate of California cannot be overlooked. The Los Angeles metropolitan area had 17 PPOs in various stages of operation and development, while the San Francisco area reported 11. San Diego had 4 preferred arrangements and San Jose 3. Only five other metro regions in the U.S. reported three or more PPOs: Denver, Miami, Chicago, Washington, D.C., and Cleveland.

The development of PPOs has not been random and appears to be closely related to the existence of certain important community indicators and health care system characteristics. The most fundamental requirement for the development of preferred panel programs is a suitable legal and legislative environ-

Table 3-1 Preferred Provider Organizations by Major Metropolitan Area as of November 1983

Metropolitan Area	State	Number PPOs
Birmingham	AL	1
Huntsville	AL	1
Little Rock	AR	1
Phoenix	AZ	2
Mesa	AZ	1
Tucson	AZ	1
Anaheim-Santa Ana-Garden Grove	CA	2
Bakersfield	CA	1
Fresno	CA	1
Los Angeles	CA	17
Oxnard-Simi Valley-Ventura	CA	2
Sacramento	CA	2
Salinas-Seaside-Monterey	CA	1
San Diego	CA	4
San Francisco-Oakland	CA	11
San Jose	CA	3
Santa Barbara	CA	1
Santa Maria-Lompoc-Santa Rosa	CA	1
Stockton	CA	1
Denver-Boulder	CO	6
Colorado Springs	CO	1
Washington	DC	4
Jacksonville	FL	2
Miami	FL	4
Ft. Lauderdale-Gainesville	FL	1
Hollywood	FL	
Tampa-St. Petersburg	FL	1
Atlanta	GA	2
Columbus	GA	1
Champaign-Urbana	IL	2
Chicago	IL	3
Gary-Hammond-East Chicago	IN	1
Des Moines	IA	2
Lexington-Fayette	KY	1
Louisville	KY	1
New Orleans	LA	2
Baltimore	MD	3
Boston	MA	1
W. Springfield	MA	1
Worcester	MA	1
Minneapolis-St. Paul	MN	2
Jackson	MS	2
Kansas City	MO	2
Reno	NV	1

Table 3-1 continued

Metropolitan Area	State	Number PPOs
Newark	NJ	1
Nassau-Suffolk	NY	3
Winston-Salem	NC	1
Cincinnati	OH	2
Cleveland	OH	5
Columbus	OH	1
Youngstown	OH	1
Warren	OH	1
Tulsa	OK	2
Portland	OR	1
Philadelphia	PA	2
Salt Lake City	UT	1
Richmond	VA	1
Roanoke	VA	1
Madison	WS	2
Milwaukee	WS	2

ment. These matters are discussed in Chapter 10. It is appropriate to note at this juncture only that legislative barriers to the establishment of preferred provider organizations do exist in certain states and these have a definite detrimental influence.[2]

In those states where legislative barriers do not exist, or are minimal, several characteristics seem to point to the overall potential for emergence of successful PPOs. As indicated in Exhibit 3-1, these include the growth rate and cosmopolitan nature of a population, its age, unemployment rates, increasing levels of employee cost sharing (for health coverage), the presence of significant levels of self-funding, business coalition activity, the existence of alternative delivery systems (particularly health maintenance organizations), a surplus of physician manpower, excess hospital beds and low hospital occupancies, and geographically proximate hospitals exhibiting a lengthy continuum of cost of care.

Demographics

Growing populations demand increasing access to medical services and an expansion of those services. New physicians migrate to growth regions. At the same time, population growth and migration suggest the presence of population groups with no, or limited, physician bonds. As a population grows and as new residents and new physicians move into a particular community, there is a decrease in the aggregate commitment level of the population to individual

Exhibit 3-1 Community Characteristics Encouraging PPO Development

Characteristic	Influence
Rapidly growing population or population with significant in- and outmigration	New community residents have no commitment to individual providers.
Relatively young population	Provider/patient relationships are less developed than with older populations.
High unemployment	Unemployment reduces physician and hospital utilization because of benefits loss.
Growing levels of employee cost sharing	100 percent of medical bills offers no incentive for use of a preferred panel; employee cost sharing does, however.
Corporate/labor union self-funding	Purchasers experience risk directly and seek ways to minimize it.
Business coalition utilization and cost reporting systems	Provider concern about the price of services is significantly greater than in areas with no reporting systems.
HMO/alternative delivery system growth	The market shares of traditional providers are adversely affected.
Surplus of physicians	Physicians are more willing to compete for patients on the basis of price.
Excess hospital beds and low hospital occupancies	Hospitals are willing to compete on basis of price to attract patients.
Close proximity of institutions providing similar quality of care	Institutional competitiveness is enhanced.
A lengthy continuum of low-cost to high-cost facilities	Purchaser price consciousness is expanded by the recognition of lower-cost, quality facilities.

providers. In such an environment, as was the case in Denver, Colorado, emerging preferred provider organizations face less resistance. Marketing of the preferred provider organization becomes much easier and the potential for success is enhanced by further population growth and migration.

In a similar manner, young populations can also be expected to have fewer and weaker bonds to individual physicians. The relative healthiness of the 16 to 45-year-old population, which predominates the U.S. workforce, precludes as frequent contact with the medical care system as more aged populations. Communities with a disproportionate age structure, characterized by large numbers of persons in this age group, have population bases less restricted by past physician preferences.

Employment

Unemployment levels serve to further enhance the probability of alternative delivery system growth. Significant unemployment levels result in the eventual loss of insurance coverage by unemployed persons. Loss of health insurance contributes to the reduction of both inpatient and outpatient medical utilization. Areas experiencing unusually high unemployment rates in times of less prosperous local economic conditions can be expected to experience reduced utilization. An overview study of the Cincinnati metropolitan area in 1983, for example, pinpointed substantial reductions in hospital utilization per 1,000 population attributed by local experts to a temporary economic slump. Such utilization reductions stimulate health providers to affiliate with alternative delivery systems.

High unemployment also contributes to the furtherance of an environment conducive to PPO development when the unemployment is primarily within a few select industries. The economic pressures created within the affected industries mandate that all available cost-cutting techniques be employed. This leads ultimately to increased pressure on employee groups and labor unions to accept greater employee cost sharing. The result is a change in employee health benefits that reduces utilization, heightening provider competition for a shrinking patient base and provider interest in PPO participation.

Cost Sharing

McClure, Enthoven, Ginsburg, and many others have advocated for several years that health coverage include sizable employee cost sharing.[3] These national policy analysts recognize, as others have, that the lack of economic incentives associated with full-pay insurance coverage creates no motivation for employees to assume a posture of prudent buying. In communities that have experienced rapid growth in employee cost sharing, like Colorado Springs, Colorado, the PPO movement has been facilitated. As employees and their dependents become financially responsible for certain appropriate portions of their medical care, the economic incentives (and disincentives) encourage the development or use of preferred panels that are available.

Self-Funding

The corporate assumption of risk represents another factor that positively influences preferred panel development, just as does employee assumption of risk through increased cost sharing. When purchasers abandon traditional insurance coverage for the benefits of self-funded arrangements, they experience quite directly the financial risk that previously had been shifted to their insurance company. The acceptance and stark recognition of this risk has done two things. First, it has awakened many corporate officials to the unusual incentives inherent in the health care financing system. In particular, those who have pursued self-funding observe quite quickly that the cost-based reimbursement system for hospitals and the fee-for-service arrangement for physicians is little more than a "cost-plus" contract offering few incentives for efficiency. The natural path taken upon such realization is one of applying common business principles to the purchase of health care services. Good businesses do not use on a frequent basis cost-plus contracting. Rather, they seek to acquire the highest quality product for the lowest reasonable price.

The existence of self-funding seems to have produced the same kind of business sense with respect to health care. Self-funding makes a purchaser aware of deficiencies in the way that services have been purchased in the past, and strongly encourages novel approaches. The preferred provider organization has served as one of the approaches that most closely parallels the business experience of many corporations and similar purchasers.

Coalitions

The existence and aggressiveness of community-based health coalitions further contribute to a conducive environment for the design and development of preferred provider organizations. Business coalitions contribute to this environment in several ways. Coalition activity heightens provider awareness about corporate and purchaser interest in controlling medical expenditures.[4] Coalitions have also undertaken certain cost-containment programs that have offered providers a glimpse of the future. Utilization control projects such as that initiated by San Diego's Employer Health Cost Coalition and Cleveland's Coalition on Health Care Cost Effectiveness have heightened provider competitiveness by reducing utilization levels for participating employers. After one year Pacific Southwest Airways, a major employer in the San Diego area, has reported a 10 percent reduction in hospital days per 1,000 employees (and dependents) as the result of preadmission certification and length of stay control programs initiated for employers in that city.[5]

Also, competition among hospitals has been boosted by the publication of hospital-specific average length of stay and charge information in some communities.

Coalitions, both by their presence and their individual activities, have subtly, and in some cases boldly, articulated purchaser commitment to cost containment and price competition. In those communities where active coalition activity has occurred, this message has served to enhance the evolution of select provider contracting opportunities.

Alternate Delivery Systems

The existence and growth of alternative delivery systems, in particular health maintenance organizations, has been discussed earlier. Health maintenance organizations have successfully competed with traditional providers for patients and have created appropriate concerns that future market share reductions might occur. The preferred provider organization is viewed by traditional providers as one way to combat the growing "menace" of prepaid programs.

The growing surplus of physicians in select metropolitan areas has uniformly encouraged preferred provider arrangements. Projections that such physician surpluses will only increase in decades to come has presented traditional fee-for-service providers with a set of new incentives to consider affiliation with systems like PPOs.

Hospital Activity

Communities experiencing excess hospital beds or low hospital occupancies further stimulate PPO activity. Inpatient acute care facilities with unused and costly capacity, or those faced with chronically low occupancies, have compelling financial incentives to pursue PPO development or involvement. Studies of communities with excess beds and minimal occupancies have noted the willingness of inpatient facilities to accept discounts from health maintenance organizations in return for increased patient volume and, therefore, a larger base of revenue.[6] The experience of HMO negotiation with hospitals confronting these problems is being repeated with preferred provider organizations. Ironically, though, low occupancy facilities may or may not be the ones with which PPOs actually contract. Aetna's CHOICE program can be described as a health care alliance among an insurance company, two hospitals, and the facilities' medical staff. The suburban Chicago program has contracted with two teaching facilities, which, as of 1983, operated at occupancy rates approximating 90 percent. Aetna officials consider occupancy pressure to be a beneficial force which continually ensures that inappropriate admissions and lengths of stay are rare occurrences.

Range of Facilities

Last, an extensive continuum of low-cost to high-cost facilities serves as an open invitation for purchasers to seek reductions in overall medical expenditures through buying decisions. The PPO is a logical vehicle.

There are other characteristics that may themselves contribute to the growth of preferred provider arrangements at the community level. Those mentioned, however, represent the major indicators of PPO activity. When several or all of these conditions are present, the probability of intense health care competition and the growth of preferred provider arrangements is all but ensured.

SPONSORSHIP AND LEGAL STRUCTURE

"If you've seen one PPO, you've seen one PPO." So goes a statement attributed to an East Coast professional involved in PPO development. The comment accurately describes the unusual variety of shapes and configurations that these entities assume. They can be established under the sponsorship of several different groups, incorporated under a variety of for-profit, not-for-profit, and joint venture models; and be linked contractually, and to different degrees, with numerous provider, purchaser, administrative, and other participants. The American Medical Care and Review Association has identified 15 different varieties of sponsorship.[7] This includes sponsorship by physician groups, individual hospitals, joint ventures by physicians and hospitals, insurance carriers of various sorts, prepaid health maintenance organizations, third party administrators, and others. Table 3-2 expands and updates the number and sponsorship of preferred provider organizations in operation and planning stages identified by the American Medical Care and Review Association in its Winter 1984 directory.

Physicians to date are the largest sponsoring group for preferred arrangements. Twenty-three percent of PPOs have been or are being established by physician groups. Joint physician/hospital programs account for an additional 16 percent. Thus, physicians are involved in the sponsorship of almost one-half of all preferred provider organizations. Individual hospitals and hospital groups sponsored 9 percent of all preferred arrangements.

In her examination of the California PPO "experiment," Trauner combined sponsorship and legal status in her classification of preferred provider arrange-

Table 3-2 Number of Preferred Provider Organizations, by Sponsorship, Fall 1983

Sponsorship	Number	Percentage
Physician	30	23
Hospital	12	9
Physician/Hospital	21	16
Blue Cross/Blue Shield Plan	4	3
Foundation for Medical Care	6	5
Blue Cross Plan	1	1
Blue Shield Plan	2	2
Insurance Carrier	10	8
Investor	9	7
IPA/HMO	4	3
Third Party Administrator	7	5
HMO	1	1
IPA	3	2
Employer Group	1	1
Consortium	1	1
Other	16	13
TOTAL	128	100

ments.[8] Three basic types were described: provider-based programs, payor-sponsored PPOs, and PPOs established by third party organizations.

THE PREFERRED PROVIDER ORGANIZATION AND OTHER FINANCING AND HEALTH CARE DELIVERY ARRANGEMENTS

An understanding of the preferred provider arrangement can be facilitated by comparing the PPO with traditional forms of insurance as well as with other alternative delivery models. Table 3-3 offers such a comparison, examining critical issues associated with (1) the assumption of risk, (2) the manner in which providers are paid under differing arrangements, (3) the existence of incentives for the use of selected providers, and (4) the extent of control exercised over the practice patterns of providers.

Traditional Insurance and the PPO

In the traditional insurance setting, the purchaser of care pays the insurer to assume the risk of care that may be required and ultimately rendered to those persons for which the purchaser has a benefits responsibility. The insurer becomes responsible for paying providers (except for copayments and deductibles). Payment is frequently on a fee-for-service basis. No real incentives exist for consumers to select efficient providers; furthermore, it is virtually impossible for consumers to have a knowledge base sufficient enough to make such selections prospectively. The traditional insurance environment offers virtually no control over the practice patterns of individual practitioners, with one notable exception. Certain insurance carriers and/or their clients may have agreements with private utilization review organizations to conduct preadmission certification, concurrent length of stay review, and other forms of utilization control.

When a traditional insurer adds a preferred provider option, the insurer still retains the risk that has been transferred to the insurer by the first-line purchaser through the payment of a premium. Again, the insurer is responsible for paying providers. The existence of the preferred panel arrangement, however, suggests that the fee-for-service payment has been prospectively negotiated and may have been discounted; also, insurance subscribers have clearly defined incentives for the use of the select panel of providers. These incentives shape consumer purchasing behavior yet are not as strong as those found in arrangements such as the exclusive provider organization and health maintenance organization. Strong controls over the practice patterns of providers may exist if aggressive utilization controls are part of the PPO.

Table 3-3 A Comparison of Health Care Financing/Delivery Models

Health care models	Who assumes risk?	Who pays providers and how?	Do incentives exist for the use of select providers?	What degree of control is exercised over provider practice patterns?
Traditional Insurance	Insurer (employee or union trust fund pays premium)	Insurer; fee for service	No	None
Traditional Insurance with PPO	Insurer (employer or union trust fund pays premium)	Insurer; prospectively negotiated, discounted fee for service	Limited	Strong, for PPO participating providers
Self-Funded Organization	Employer or union trust fund	Employer or union trust fund; fee for service	No	None
Self-Funded Organization with PPO	Employer or union trust fund	Employer or union trust fund; prospectively negotiated, discounted fee for service	Limited	Strong, for PPO participating providers
Self-Funded Organization with EPO	Employer or union trust fund	Employer or union trust fund; prospectively negotiated, discounted fee for service	Extremely strong	Strong
Health Care Alliance	Insurer (employer/subscribing group pays premium)	Insurer; typically fee for service	Extremely strong	Limited
Health Maintenance Organization (HMO)	HMO (employer/subscribing group pays premium)	HMO; physicians frequently paid on capitation basis	Extremely strong	Strong
Independent Practice Associations (IPA)	IPA (employer/subscribing group pays premium)	IPA; physician paid on capitation or fee for service basis	Extremely strong	Limited to strong

Self-Funding and the PPO

A self-funding arrangement, whether undertaken by an employer or union trust fund, has characteristics similar to the traditional insurance (only) option. The major exception is that the employer or union trust fund assumes the financial risk, or the majority of that risk, rather than transferring it to an insurer. Second, the self-funding entity pays providers either directly or through a third party administrator. Incentives for the use of a select panel of providers do not exist. There is no control over the practice patterns of providers who render care to persons covered by the self-funding arrangement.

The addition of a preferred panel does not alter the element of risk or the responsibility for paying providers. It does, however, change the way providers are paid, from routine fee-for-service to prospectively negotiated (probably discounted) fee-for-service arrangements. The addition of utilization review establishes a strong element of control over providers in the panel and there are financial incentives for employees or union members to use the preferred panel.

If the preferred panel becomes an exclusive panel, one very substantial alteration takes place. As the name implies, an exclusive provider organization (EPO) is a delivery system in which care is paid for only when provided by the limited and select group of physicians and hospitals. Thus, central to the EPO are extremely strong financial incentives for the consumers to use the exclusive panel. The failure to use this panel results in financial responsibility for total payment (or almost total payment) by the consumer. Cubic Corporation is a self-funded West Coast company that offers its employees several health insurance options. In July 1983, the company added an exclusive provider organization to coverage options offered to its San Diego-based employee group. The EPO costs the employee less than the other options. Employees must receive medical care from The Scripps Clinic, its medical staff, and a limited number of private practice physicians/groups that have contracted with The Scripps Clinic program.

The Health Care Alliance

The insurance equivalent to a self-funded EPO is the health care alliance. The health care alliance is a medical delivery model in which an insurer contracts with a select group of providers and markets care by the group to purchasers, who pay a premium reflecting the efficiency of the exclusive panel. The health care alliance, exemplified by Aetna's CHOICE in Chicago, includes very strong economic incentives for consumers to use the preferred panel, is based on a traditional fee-for-service payment, and generally has a less rigorous set of utilization control procedures than those that accompany preferred provider arrangements.

HMOs and IPAs

Health maintenance organizations and independent practice associations vary from the above arrangements in (1) the placement of risk and (2) the way physicians are paid. The HMO or IPA entity assumes financial risk for care rendered to enrollees. At the same time, the entity frequently places some of that risk directly on the providers of care. Financial risk is transferred to providers through the use of capitation payments, that is, lump sum payments for each enrollee for which providers fund any and all care required. The capitation payment is age and sex adjusted. Fee-for-service payment may be used for certain kinds of specialists and for consultations beyond the boundaries of the HMO or IPA, but the central characteristic of these organizations is the placement of financial incentives on physicians to provide efficient, cost-conscious care. Consumer incentives are substantial. The use of non-HMO or non-IPA physicians results in direct consumer responsibility for incurred medical bills. Utilization controls are notoriously strong in both HMOs and, to a lesser degree, IPAs.

PPO adoption of certain operating procedures used by HMOs/IPAs tends to blur the difference between these delivery systems, particularly from the provider and patient perspective. PPOs adopting case management and primary care physician capitation payment systems, in combination with strong utilization controls, closely approximate the incentive and operational characteristics of prepaid alternate delivery systems. For PPO consumers, restrictions placed on the use of select providers and the financial penalties imposed for not using the select panel (particularly in an exclusive provider arrangement) parallel consumer experiences in HMOs and IPAs. San Diego's Cubic/Scripps Plan, the EPO mentioned earlier, offers an example of the "delivery system blur" taking place between HMOs/IPAs and PPOs. Cubic employees electing the EPO health benefit option are covered by the plan only when Scripps Clinic, its physicians, and a designated group of other physicians are used. Like a staff model HMO, EPO enrollees must use this numerically limited number of providers. PPO enrollees using nonaffiliated providers assume total financial responsibility for the cost of care (except in emergency situations).

The Cubic/Scripps Plan also employs a capitation payment system for primary care practitioners while paying specialists on a fee-for-service basis. Again, from the observation point of the primary care practitioner, the Cubic/Scripps Plan mirrors an IPA-type HMO while, for the specialist, it assumes the more general appearance of a PPO.

From PPO to HMO

It can be expected that as preferred provider organizations gain operating experience and develop the capability to accurately forecast financial risks, increasing movement toward HMO-like operations will occur. Conceptually, there is good reason for this. If one examines the short, hasty development of preferred provider organizations, a basic evolutionary path appears. Early PPO initiators offered discounts but frequently lacked aggressive utilization and quality control mechanisms. These preferred provider organizations represented marketing frameworks for the brokers who initiated them or the institutions that developed them. The second evolutionary phase was the addition of aggressive utilization review and controls. Utilization review was added as an important feature designed to increase purchaser interest. As of 1983, a third evolutionary phase began. It is designed to restructure the incentive and financing aspects of medical care, rather than merely offer discounts and place practice restrictions on providers. This third phase is characterized by (1) risk-sharing payment mechanisms (capitated physician case management approaches, hospital payment systems based on per diems, payment per confinement, and DRG-type reimbursement) and (2) other financial incentive systems for physicians and hospitals.

This evolution, from a marketing orientation to one that includes a restructuring of provider incentives, should continue for two reasons. First, purchasers of care are adamant in their desire to share the financial risks of care with consumers and providers. Cost sharing at the employee level, and the implementation of financial incentives for providers through a PPO, begin to meet these purchaser needs. Preferred provider arrangements intent on successfully meeting this market demand will move toward increasing risk-sharing arrangements. Second, visionary providers recognize that capitation and per diem/per case payment methods can generate healthy profits not necessarily available through traditional fee-for-service and cost-based reimbursement. Efficient providers will view participation in such payment methods as an opportunity rather than a risk. One can expect that efficient PPOs and their associated providers will pursue these opportunities as they gain increasing experience with the costs of operation and the economic implications of greater risk assumption.

The relationship between health maintenance organizations and preferred provider organizations, and the potential for PPOs to evolve into HMO-like structures, can also be viewed in a reverse fashion. PPOs will not only increasingly adopt HMO-type characteristics; HMOs/IPAs have and will increasingly develop PPO products. One example of this is the AV-MED Preferred Provider Organization in Miami, Florida. AV-MED PPO is a new product line offered by an existing HMO. AV-MED Health Maintenance Organization has been in operation for a number of years. It is a state-certified, federally qualified HMO with over 42,000 members. It is the largest individual practice association type HMO in the southeastern United States. AV-MED currently provides its enrollees with access to over 1,000 private practitioners and 25 hospitals in the Miami metropolitan area.

The number of HMO/IPA organizations that have established preferred panel arrangements is limited. The Winter 1984 *Directory of Preferred Provider Organizations* published by the American Medical Care and Review Association noted only two, including AV-MED. However, there appears to be at least three primary reasons these prepaid delivery systems can be expected to spin off preferred provider arrangements as a separate product marketed to the purchaser community. First, these organizations have already established panels of physicians and hospitals, and contractual relationships with these providers. Accordingly, much of the difficulty of establishing a PPO is nonexistent. Second, HMOs and IPAs have established data systems for monitoring practice patterns of providers and for conducting utilization review activities. The high cost of establishing these has, then, been incurred already. Last, HMOs or IPAs have the ability to specify the efficiency characteristics of providers as a condition for participation in the preferred panel. Well-organized delivery systems have hospital- and physician-specific capabilities that allow a rigorous level of efficiency screening.

Part of the reason few HMOs have actively established preferred arrangements may relate to an August 1983 issuance from the Office of Health Maintenance Organizations, U.S. Department of Health and Human Services. The purpose of that issuance was to clarify for federally qualified health maintenance organizations whether federal law and regulations allow these organizations to establish preferred provider arrangements. The Office noted that:

> Title XIII of the Public Health Service Act (the Act) and its implementing regulations do not permit a federally qualified HMO, itself, to indemnify its members for basic health services the member receives from physicians who have no affiliation with the HMO or . . . (other) medical group through which it provides such services . . . Since an indemnity arrangement would result in physician services (which are basic health services) being provided by a non-affiliated physician in a circumstance not covered by one of the permitted exceptions, we have concluded that such an arrangement does not meet the requirements for federally qualified HMOs.[9]

The guidance offered by the Office of Health Maintenance Organizations strongly suggested that HMO enrollees could not receive services outside of the HMO except for certain emergencies through a PPO-type arrangement. This, however, does not appear to be the fundamental issue associated with HMO/PPO relationships. A more salient matter appears to be whether an HMO, using its contracts with physicians and hospitals, can market this set of providers as a preferred panel and be paid on a fee-for-service basis for services rendered by the panel. The Office of Health Maintenance Organizations suggested, again, that this was probably inconsistent with legislative intent. The Office noted:

> This basis for the conclusion . . . is reinforced by the following interpretation of the intent of Congress and section 1311. That section

exempts qualified HMOs from the initial capitalization and financial reserve requirements of state insurance laws. Had Congress contemplated that an HMO engage in insurance activities—and indemnifying a member is an insurance function—it would seem reasonable that Congress would not have provided this exemption. Said differently, a qualified HMO may not take advantage of that status to escape state regulation of an insurance function that Congress contemplated the HMO would not undertake.[10]

This advice, however, is inconsistent with the experience of most preferred provider organizations, which are presently not considered as having indemnity arrangements, and which are not regulated by state insurance laws.

The August 1983 issuance leaves some room for PPO participation, though it notes that the guidelines do not preclude an HMO from setting up a separate corporation to engage in PPO activity.

Regardless of the advice presented to date, it appears that PPOs will face increasing demands both internally and from external sources to adopt HMO-like risk-sharing features. Conversely, HMOs will consider the potential of PPO product development. Perhaps the most critical issue for HMOs will not be technical in nature or even regulatory; rather, it will relate to political difficulties concerning the IPA model HMOs, which, by necessity, may wish to open the PPO product only to the most efficient physicians. Many IPAs will have little technical difficulty in doing this since they have well-established data review systems for identifying the efficient. The selection of an efficient elite, who form the core of a PPO product, introduces the immediate risk of alienating other physicians participating in the IPA. One Ohio-based IPA has indicated this as the primary reason it may not develop a PPO product.

THE IMPACT OF PREFERRED PROVIDER ARRANGEMENTS

Preferred provider arrangements have been examined from a variety of angles to this point. But all the studying, analysis, and review of PPO characteristics has little meaning if, in aggregate, they do not produce the benefits expected from them. Most of the expected impact is financial in nature. Some is not. The purpose of this section is to explore reports and evidence suggesting that PPOs influence, both positively and negatively, the environments in which they exist.

Conceptually, there is every reason to expect constructive economic outcomes for purchasers, physicians, hospitals, and consumers. The inclusion of a variety of cost-containing features—utilization review, provider selection and termination criteria, discounts, alternative payment arrangements—hint strongly at the ability of these competitive medical plans to benefit purchasers. Incentives encouraging consumers to use preferred panels seem to portend positive experiences for consumers and providers as well.

The ultimate and indeed short-term issue for the PPO movement is a simple one: Do PPOs actually restrain medical inflation? If they do not, the movement is doomed to failure because, simply, there will be no purchaser for the PPO product. In examining the financial impact of PPOs, this question must be addressed first.

Much of the information included in the following sections is anecdotal in nature. Few preferred provider organizations have a track record that is sufficiently lengthy to provide conclusive evidence that PPOs do, in the long term, produce substantial impact upon participants. The cases illustrated here are simply examples of what can be achieved in the short term by well-planned and organized PPOs. One may or may not wish to draw inferences for the long term from them. One thing is certain, however—without a short term there can be no long term.

The Impact on Purchasers

The expected and reported impact of PPOs can be described from several perspectives: reductions in utilization levels and lengths of stay, discount levels, and/or estimated dollar savings. Table 3-4 offers a representative sample of impacts attributed to and expected from preferred provider arrangements.

Tulsa's CompMed is a hospital-affiliated PPO that, because of its hospital association, has been able to compare the utilization and cost experience of PPO enrollees with that of non-PPO participants. This comparison has been further enhanced by a diagnosis-specific data system. In the first several months of operation in 1983, CompMed found that the average length of stay for PPO users was .7 to .3 of one day less, and 8 percent less costly than comparable hospital populations. Martin E. Segal has reported a 12 percent length of stay reduction for its clients whose employees and union members have used preferred provider panels.

The Lutheran Hospital Society of Southern California was one of the early entrants into the West Coast PPO market, initially making its facilities and physicians available to employees of the multihospital chain. By 1982, the Society was reporting that hospital days used per 1,000 employees were estimated to be 18 percent less than the experience of hospital employees throughout the state (650 versus 800 patient days per 1,000 population). Lutheran Society officials estimated that the introduction of the preferred provider concept was saving the Society's self-funded health benefit plan an estimated $300,000 to $400,000 annually for its 5,000 covered employees.

Some preferred provider arrangements have been able to identify anticipated cost savings for purchasers in advance of the operation of their programs. Two of the best examples are United PPO, Inc., and The Physicians' Alliance for Medical Excellence.

Table 3-4 Impact of PPOs on Purchasers: Reported and Expected

Purchaser Group	Reported or Expected Impact	Source
PPO participants, Tulsa, Oklahoma	The average length of stay was reduced .7–.3 of a day for PPO patients. PPO patients experience costs that are 8 percent less costly than for comparable diagnoses.	CompMed, Tulsa, Oklahoma (personal communication).
PPO subscribing groups, San Diego, California	Average negotiated per diem discount approaches 30 percent.	San Diego PPO, Inc., San Diego, California (personal communication).
Security Pacific Corporation, Los Angeles, California	One hospital provides discounts of $600 per day for PPO patients. Estimated annual savings may be as high as $800,000 when PPO participation commences (25,000 employees) in late 1983.	R.L. Rundle, *Business Insurance* (May 30, 1983): 16.
Blue Cross of California, Oakland, California	A premium reduction of 10 percent due to the Prudent Buyer Plan is the goal.	S. Viau, *PPOs: State of the Art*, 1983, p. 27.
Lutheran Hospital Society of Southern California (self-insured corporation)	Save $300,000 to $400,000 annually due to PPO for employees (5,000 employees).	A. Kornblum, *Business Week* (September 20, 1982): 117.
Self-funded corporations and labor union trust funds using Martin E. Segal Company, Denver, Colorado, as benefits consultant	PPO utilization controls have reduced patient days per 1,000 employees to 650. The comparable figure for hospital employees statewide is 800 patient days per 1,000 employees. Savings in 1981 were $330,000 on $4.5 million in hospital claims.	D. Gibbons, *Medical World News* (February 28, 1983): 64. D. Gibbons, *Medical World News* (February 28, 1983): 64.
Individual purchasers subscribing to PPO	Based on 1982 Blue Cross/Blue Shield data, the total hospital cost per case for PPO member physicians was more than 15 percent less than peer averages; average length of stay was 11 percent less.	Physicians' Alliance, Lexington, Kentucky (personal communication).

Table 3-4 continued

Purchaser Group	Reported or Expected Impact	Source
Union members, Denver, Colorado	Union trust fund payments for union members/dependents who sought care from preferred providers increased only 5 percent during 1981. Nationally, health inflation was about 15 percent.	S.B. Barger, *The Bulletin of the New York City Association of Life Underwriters*, 62, no. 4 (November 1982): 37.
	Physician fee schedules rose only 5 percent in the 1981–82 yearly negotiation.	D. Lefton, *American Medical News* (May 7, 1982): 21.
Rohr Industries, Chula Vista, California	1982 savings approached $300,000. These were obtained through negotiated hospital discounts only. Future PPO involvement is expected to save 15 percent.	*Coalition Report*, 2, no. 3 (May 1983): 1. Rohr Industries (personal communication).
Groups contracting with California foundations for medical care, California	Dollars not paid out (because of coordination of benefits, peer review, maximum allowable charges, etc.) equaled 28 percent of initial billed charges on statewide basis for 1982. Individual foundations for medical care reported savings of 21 percent to 31 percent for same time period.	United Foundations for Medical Care, San Francisco, California (marketing/PR materials).
Clients of Martin E. Segal Company, Denver, Colorado	PPOs associated with Martin E. Segal and Company have reduced average length of stay for Segal clients by 12 percent.	*Hospital Peer Review*, 7, no. 5 (May 1982): 56.
State of California, Medi-Cal program	California's select hospital contracting program expects to save $225 million in its first year; an additional $150 million could be saved by more aggressive contracting.	*Health Policy Week*, 12, no. 22 (June 6, 1983): 3.
Clients of California Preferred Professionals (CPP), Los Angeles, California	Through utilization controls, CPP estimates that 22–40 percent can be achieved off a purchaser's present health care expenditures.	S. Viau, *PPOs: State of the Art*, 1983, p. 26.
Unnamed Insurance Carrier, (associated with Med Network), California	1981 costs for Med Network clients were 23 percent less than standard indemnity plan clients.	S. Viau, *PPOs: State of the Art*, 1983, p. 32.

Comprehensive-type foundations affiliated with United PPO's parent, the United Foundations for Medical Care, employ cost-containment features similar to those found in PPOs (aggressive utilization review, competitive charge structures, patient insulation from nonreimbursed fees, etc.). One exception is that until July 1983 the foundations did not have negotiated discounts/competitive fee structures with hospitals. A 1982 analysis of these PPO-like entities concluded that dollars not paid out because of cost-containment features approximated 28 percent of initial billed charges for foundations in the state of California. The four foundations from which this estimate was derived reported individual savings ranging from 21 percent to 31 percent. Such savings, prior to hospital contracting, hint at the potential these organizations possess.

The Physicians' Alliance is a full-fledged preferred provider entity. Its physician selection process, summarized in a later section, requires that inpatient practice efficiency data maintained by Blue Cross/Blue Shield of Kentucky be made available for examination prior to acceptance for participation in this physician-sponsored program.

The organization has determined that its physicians have practice patterns that are 15 percent less expensive than comparable medical professionals. Such advance knowledge of the PPO's performance has not gone unnoticed by purchaser groups in the Lexington, Kentucky, region that are served by the Physicians' Alliance.

Purchaser cost savings approaching 25 percent have also been reported by West Coast purchasers. A California insurance carrier that offered groups access to the preferred provider panel organized by the third party administrator AdMar reported that for 1981 preferred panel users experienced costs 23 percent lower than standard indemnity plan subscribers who did not use the panel providers.

A variety of expected purchaser cost savings are highlighted in Table 3-4. Perhaps the most notable are the estimates reported by Viau for California Preferred Professionals (CPP). This PPO anticipates that purchaser health expenses can be reduced 22 to 40 percent depending on the breadth and type of utilization controls employed.

Though purchasers consider hospital discounts to be only a very small portion of overall cost savings, fee/charge reductions must nevertheless be viewed by those who pay for medical services as another area of favorable financial outcome. Generally, discounts from billed charges do not exceed 15 percent, with many being closer to the 5 to 10 percent range.

Some very notable exceptions to this do exist, though. In the highly competitive San Diego hospital marketplace, average discounts from historic per diem costs are informally said to be in the 30 percent range; one hospital is reportedly discounting services to PPO patients by $600 a day. Obviously, this facility is at the high end of the $400 to $1,100 per day San Diego hospital cost continuum.

Of course, hospital discounts in and of themselves do not necessarily indicate cost restraint. Purchasers are acutely aware that a 20 percent discount off the price of a commodity that is 50 percent costlier than comparable products is not much of a cost savings.

The Impact of PPOs on Physicians

The impact PPOs have on physicians can take several forms. The most obvious concern (1) the extent to which PPOs produce new business, (2) the limits and/ or fee discounts associated with PPO participation, (3) cash flow improvement resulting from rapid claims payment, and (4) the degree to which PPOs actually restrict participation by questionable or inefficient physicians. The inability of PPOs to accomplish the first three affect their ability to consistently attract and retain competent medical professionals. The failure to successfully conduct the fourth has the long-term potential to retard the competitiveness and viability of an individual PPO.

The extent to which any of these impacts has been quantitatively observed in PPOs is particularly limited. Table 3-5, however, offers a few of the quantitative observations and reports of the impact on physicians.

Two estimates from different areas of the U.S. suggest that the offering of a PPO option results in high usage of the preferred panel by consumers. Ohio Health Choice Plan is a statewide, franchised PPO with about 10 hospitals linked to its program. Most groups offering Ohio Health Choice pay fully for care rendered by the physician panel but cover only 80 percent of costs when services are from nonpanel practitioners. This level of financial incentive has been adequate enough to produce a panel use rate of 80 percent; that is, subscribers use the preferred panel and take advantage of its financial advantages 80 percent of the time. West Coast use estimates have been smaller but still impressive. A 1982 examination found preferred provider organizations experiencing a 50 percent panel use rate.

The implications of these subjective findings are of serious interest to physicians considering PPO involvement, for they hint at the competitive success of the preferred arrangement. The impact on any one practitioner's practice will, naturally, vary, depending on many factors. Anecdotal information suggests that physicians can expect PPO patients to account for 5 to 10 percent of their total patient volume, though an important question must be raised about the percent of new, compared to previous, patients. Again, anecdotal information from Mountain Medical Affiliates indicates that half of all PPO patients may be new; Mountain Medical physicians have reported, for example, that PPO patients account for 5 percent of some individual practices but only 2½ percent are actually new patients. The remaining 2½ percent represent conversion patients. It is interesting to note also that a distinct minority of Mountain Medical phy-

Table 3-5 Impact of PPOs on Physicians: Reported and/or Expected

Reported/Expected Impact	*Source*
Once a PPO is offered to an employee group, 50 percent of that group will use it. This depends, obviously, on the level of incentives. For highly concentrated groups of employees, the impact on physicians and hospitals could be significant. (Los Angeles, California)	*FAH Review* (July/August 1982): 24.
Once a PPO is offered to an employee group, 80 percent of that group used the preferred panel. (Cleveland, Ohio)	Ohio Health Choice Plan (personal communication).
Some physicians have seen as much as a 50 percent increase in their patient load due to PPOs. These are the exception, though, not the rule. (Denver, Colorado)	D.L. Gibbons, *Medical World News* (February 28, 1983): 61.
Physicians reported that less than 5 percent of their business was PPO patients; 2½ percent were new and resulted from the PPO. (Denver, Colorado)	D. Leffon, *American Medical News* (May 7, 1982): 21.
Physicians reported that 5 to 10 percent of practice was PPO patients. (Denver, Colorado)	D.L. Gibbons, *Medical World News* (February 28, 1983): 63.
Physician payment schedules were 80 to 85 percent of UCR. (Various cities)	Report to the Council of Medical Services to Reference Committee G. American Medical Association, 1982.
Physicians are reducing usual fee rates of from 14 to 18 percent for PPO patients. (Denver, Colorado)	D.L. Gibbons, *Medical World News* (February 28, 1983): 61.
Physician payment is based on the 50th percentile of prevailing fees. (Kansas City, Missouri)	Preferred Health Professionals, Kansas City, Missouri.
Physician payment is based at the 90th percentile of UCR. (Tulsa, Oklahoma)	CompMed, Tulsa, Oklahoma, 1983 (personal communication).
Approximately 2½ percent of physicians applying for membership in a West Coast PPO were rejected. (Los Angeles, California)	S. Viau, *PPOs: The State of the Art*, 1983, p. 25.
Physician/provider discounts may approach 20 percent.	S.B. Barger, *The Bulletin of the New York City Association of Life Underwriters* 62, no. 4 (November 1982): 37.
Under typical payment arrangements, payment to physicians may average 40 to 90 days. PPOs have reduced this to less than 10 days. (Denver, Colorado)	Martin E. Segal Company, Denver, Colorado (personal communication).
One benefits administrator reports same-day payment (i.e., payment is mailed on day bill is received). (Denver, Colorado)	Fringe Benefits Services, Denver, Colorado (personal communication).

sicians have experienced tremendous growth in patient volume as the result of PPO participation. Increases of as much as 50 percent have been identified by a small number of practitioners.

The limited conclusion that might be drawn is that physicians can indeed increase patient volume, and do so handsomely in select instances, through participation in a viable preferred panel program. Physicians experiencing sizable increases in patient volume will most likely be those who exhibit a combination of several characteristics:

- A practice location in close proximity to many groups participating in the PPO
- A relative dearth of other practitioners in the same geographical area affiliation with a specialty that is substantially underrepresented in the PPO
- A very visible professional reputation

Physicians considering PPO participation will necessarily want to assess their own particular situation and the degree to which it has similarities to these characteristics.

The observed increases in opportunity for increasing an individual physician's productivity and revenue enhancement is only partially determined by volume increases. The second major element of the revenue equation is the level of fee discount required from affiliated physicians. The issue of discounts has been one of misunderstanding and controversy; it is covered in more detail in Chapter 5. At this juncture only a few summary statements about discounts are appropriate. First, most PPOs use some tool for limiting physician payment. Discounted relative value scales and the use of less-than-full payment under UCR schedules are the most common. Second, regardless of the method used, discounts are offered. Discounts between 10 and 20 percent seem to be the most common. Exhibit 2-1 in Chapter 2 provides a glimpse of the variability in both method and level of physician reimbursement approaches. In 1982, CompMed paid physicians up to the 90th percentile of the UCR while Preferred Health Professionals pays only the 50th percentile of prevailing fees. Mountain Medical Affiliates uses a relative value scale; physicians there reduce usual fee rates from 14 to 18 percent for PPO patients.

Revenue enhancement is also a function of payment promptness. Personal communications from select PPO officials indicate that many physicians may typically wait 40 to 90 days for payment under traditional insurance reimbursement approaches. In Denver, PPO affiliation has reduced this to less than 10 days for physicians associated with PPOs used by clients of the Martin E. Segal Company. At least one third party administrator fringe benefit associate routinely issues physician reimbursement the same day that bills arrive. It is commonplace for PPOs in general to require that purchasers pay within 30, and sometimes within 15 days.

Clearly, one of the most sensitive and difficult impacts to assess is the frequency with which preferred provider arrangements limit physician participation or expel questionable practitioners previously admitted to a preferred panel network. Viau's book on PPOs mentions that one Los Angeles area organization rejects roughly 2½ percent of those physicians applying for membership.[11] On the East Coast the Greater Baltimore PPO, following an analysis of partially available physician practice information, reportedly invited only those physicians considered to be the 20 percent most efficient practitioners.

PPOs have generally avoided stringent admission efficiency criteria for two reasons. First, the quantitative data for such assessments is rarely available. Second, PPO developers have been uncomfortable over any action that might adversely alter the ability of a medical practitioner to practice his or her skill (more commonly referred to as the antitrust violation restraint of trade). Consequently the prevailing logic seems to be that "all are welcome but only the efficient may remain." Statistics on physician expulsions, should one wish to term them as such, are nonexistent. High expulsion rates might be viewed constructively. On the other hand, observers might consider such behavior indicative of poor quality and effectiveness to begin with. Obvious peril faces those organizations viewed within the latter context and, accordingly, it is not difficult to understand the reasons that preferred provider entities may choose to keep this information inaccessible.

Physicians unconcerned about PPO efficiency and billing guidelines can expect to be faced with professional irritations. Herein lies a useful and less adversarial technique PPOs can and do employ to thin the ranks of deviant professionals. Persistent professional review and gentle admonishment have been used, either consciously or unconsciously, to encourage select small numbers of physicians to remove members from the PPO.

One Denver PPO has reported in the health literature that two physicians, disgruntled with PPO utilization review and billing policies voluntarily disassociated from the organization.[12]

The Impact of PPOs on Hospitals

Hospital involvement in preferred provider arrangements may come about for numerous reasons. However, two almost universal reasons for participation are related to (1) the protection/expansion of the hospital patient base and (2) the stabilization/enhancement of an institution's total revenue position. Table 3-6 illustrates some of these.

One of the most notable and visible examples of the impact a PPO can have on a hospital's volume and revenue comes from the hospital system linked with

Table 3-6 Impact of PPOs on Hospitals: Reported and/or Expected

Hospital	Impact	Source
Baptist Medical Center, Kansas City, Missouri	Announcement of PPO development produced increase in admissions by physicians on courtesy staff interested in pursuing active staff status (a requirement for PPO participation).	Personal communication
Presbyterian/St. Luke's Medical Center, Denver, Colorado	In 1981, PPO patients accounted for 2 percent of participating hospital's revenue, equaling about $2 million. One percent of revenue came from patients attracted by the discount arrangement.	D. Lefton, *American Medical News* (May 7, 1982): 21.
	PPO participation accounted for over 4,300 patient days in 1982 and was expected to approximate 6,500 patient days in 1983. The hospital's goal is that 5 to 7 percent of revenue will come from PPO participation.	*FAH Review* (July/August 1982): 13.
Presbyterian/St. Luke's Medical Center, Denver, Colorado	During first six months of PPO operation, 45 percent of patients served had not previously used the hospital system.	*FAH Review* (July/August 1982): 31.
Physicians and hospitals participating in Far-West Administrators PPO (COMPETE), California	Reported insolvency of Far West Administrators left $11 million in unpaid physician and hospital claims.	M.L. O'Connor, *Hospital Forum* (November/December 1982): 19.

Denver's Mountain Medical Affiliates: Presbyterian/St. Luke's Medical Center. In 1981/82 hospital officials estimated that 1 percent ($1,000,000) of the hospital's revenue came from patients attracted by the discount arrangements. An additional 1 percent of revenue was generated by PPO patients but these patients used the facility because of past affiliation with the medical center and its medical staff. This revenue split is consistent with other data from the medical center indicating that during the first six months of the hospital's involvement in the PPO, 45 percent of patients served had not previously used the Presbyterian/ St. Luke's Medical Center System. The Medical Center's eventual goal is for the PPO product to generate from 5 to 7 percent of the hospital system's total revenue.

Other favorable impacts may also await facilities seeking PPO affiliation. In 1983, Baptist Medical Center in Kansas City, Missouri, initiated a PPO product called Preferred Health Professionals; only active medical staff members were eligible for membership. The requirement that active medical staff status be obtained prior to PPO participation encouraged several practitioners to alter their admission patterns to gain this status. The result was a pleasant one for the Baptist Medical Center: patient admissions increased.

Finally, there's both good news and bad news for PPO-affiliated institutions. The good news has been stated; the bad news is probably obvious to any serious student of the PPO movement: hospitals linked to financially shaky preferred provider arrangements can lose revenue. One of the most salient examples has been reported insolvency of Far West Administrators PPO (COMPETE) in California. The organization's insolvency left an estimated $11 million in unpaid physician and hospital bills. Although such failures to date have been apparently rare, they do serve the purpose of reminding all involved that PPOs are business, as well as medical, enterprises.

NOTES

1. Clearinghouse on Preferred Provider Organizations, *Directory of Preferred Provider Organizations* (Bethesda, Md.: Institute for International Initiatives, Winter 1984), i.

2. For a generic discussion of legislative and regulatory considerations, see *Hospital Council of Southern California Preferred Provider Organization Contracting Manual: Issues and Strategies* (Los Angeles: May 1983), 2-19 to 2-41. American Medical Association. "Selected Insurance Code Provisions." State Health Legislation Report. Vol. 11, No. 1, February, 1983, pp. 7–25.

3. Walter McClure, "Redesigning Benefits Stimulates Cost Consciousness," *Business and Health* (November 1983): 23–26; Walter McClure, "Implementing a Competitive Medical System Through Public Policy," *Journal of Health Politics, Policy of Law* 7, no. 1 (1982): 2–44; A.C. Enthoven, *Consumer Choice Health Plan: The Only Practical Solution to the Soaring Cost of Medical Care* (Reading, Mass.: Addison-Wesley, 1980); P.B. Ginsburg, "Altering the Tax Treatment of Employment-Based Health Plans," *Milbank Memorial Fund Quarterly* 59, no. 2 (Spring 1981): 224–255.

4. S. Brian Barger and David G. Hillman, *Future Directions in Health: A Review of Significant Trends Likely To Influence Hospital Care in the 1980s* (Cincinnati, Oh.: Morgan Bigae Institute, October 4, 1982): 13.

5. Personal communication with Robert Colasanto, Director of Insurance and Employee Benefits, Pacific Southwest Airlines, June 1983.

6. J.E. Kralewski, D.D. Countryman, and L. Pitt, "Hospital and Health Maintenance Organization Financial Agreements for Inpatient Services: A Case Study of Minneapolis/St. Paul," *Health Care Financing Review* 4, no. 4 (Summer 1983): 79–84; J.B. Christianson, "The Competitive Approach to Health Care Reform: Implications for Hospital Management," *Health Care Management Review* (Fall 1981): 7–15.

7. Clearinghouse on Preferred Provider Organizations, *Directory of Preferred Provider Organizations*, i.

8. Joan B. Trauner, *Preferred Provider Organizations: The California Experiment* (San Francisco: University of California, August 1983), 21–24.

9. F.H. Seubold, *Further Guidance on PPO Issues*, OHMO Program Information Letter 83-04, August 1983.

10. Ibid.

11. Suzanne Viau, *PPOs: The State of the Art* (Washington, D.C.: Health Publishing Ventures, 1983), 25.

12. Don L. Gibbons, "Doctors Hope Cut-Rate 'Preferred Provider' Organizations Can Fill Empty Waiting Rooms," *Medical World News* (February 28, 1983): 63.

Part II

Cost Control in Preferred Panel Arrangements

Chapter 4

Influencing Consumer Behavior: Rewarding Prudent Buying Decisions

Preferred provider organizations do not necessarily alter traditional financial incentives to providers, the exception being those instances in which some financial risk is shared through the use of per diem or per case hospital payments and capitation payments to physicians. Sufficient incentives to alter behavior do exist at the consumer level, however. A two- or three-tiered system shapes consumer selection of (1) health benefits, (2) providers, and (3) health services.

CONSUMER INCENTIVES

Health Benefits Selection

The first tier offers the consumer the availability of different health benefit or insurance options. This is often referred to in an employment setting as "dual choice." Potential health benefit choices might include an IPA model health maintenance organization, traditional coverage through a Blue Cross plan or other commercial insurer, a preferred provider organization, and/or an exclusive provider organization. Figure 4-1 illustrates a health benefits coverage "menu" composed of these four options. This example has been drawn from a West Coast high-tech company.

Consumers selecting the exclusive provider organization pay no monthly employee contribution for a family contract. The IPA model health maintenance organization, on the other hand, costs $38 per month; its potential attractiveness is enhanced because out-of-pocket contributions are virtually eliminated as long as the IPA providers render care. The traditional insurance coverage option and the PPO are provided in tandem. That is, consumers selecting the traditional insurance option continue to have the option to use the preferred panel and receive the economic benefits associated with that panel. But the ability to oscillate between unlimited provider selection on the one hand and a small subset

Figure 4-1 Employee Selection of Health Coverage and Associated Financial Consequences: An Example

Monthly Payment	Coverage Type	Financial Consequences
	IPA	• 100% Coverage • No out-of-pocket payments
$38/Month	or	
	IPA Panel Not Used	• 0% Coverage
	Traditional Insurance	• 80% Coverage and • $250 Deductible and • $3,000 Maximum out-of-pocket expenditure
$20/Month	or	
	Preferred Panel Used	• 100% Coverage • $0 Deductible • $1,000 Maximum out-of-pocket expenditure
	EPO	
$0/Month	or	
	Preferred Panel Not Used	• 0% Coverage

Employee — Coverage Selected

composed of preferred professionals on the other has financial penalties. A monthly payment of $20 is required regardless of which providers are eventually used. Also, a sizable out-of-pocket liability exists when the preferred panel is not used voluntarily for care.

The first tier of financial incentives facing the consumer, then, concerns consumer willingness to limit provider choice and/or take on greater financial responsibility for those services eventually rendered.

Provider Selection

The second tier of financial incentives comes into play when the consumer requires a medical service (Table 4-1). Under both the IPA and EPO options, the consumer is frequently given 100 percent coverage of the service as long as the panel of providers in the IPA or the exclusive provider organization is used.

If the provider in either of these benefit coverage options is not used, the consumer, in most cases, becomes financially responsible for the full cost of care rendered. The financial incentives for the use of the selected providers in both the IPA and the exclusive provider organization are significant.

The relationship between traditional insurance coverage and the preferred provider arrangement, as well as the financial incentives that encourage the use of the preferred panel, are more complex. The traditional insurance option allows care to be provided by virtually any medical professional or institution. For the privilege of such broad choice, the consumer is faced with deductibles, potentially large out-of-pocket expenses, and only an 80 percent payment level for many routine and costly services. On the other hand, the consumer minimizes, if not eliminates, these financial contributions when care is provided by the participating panel of preferred providers.

In this instance, the financial risk of the consumer closely parallels that for those persons enrolled in the exclusive provider organization. The one difference is the monthly contribution. This contribution allows the consumer to switch back and forth regularly between an unrestricted pool of health providers and the select panel. Those individuals who desire to use the select panel regularly would be best served, in this example, by enrolling in the exclusive provider organization that does not require a monthly contribution.

In her examination of California preferred provider organizations, Trauner examined the financial impact of an individual consumer decision to use, or not to use, the preferred panel of a PPO or EPO.[1] In exploring the financial impact on the consumer, three reimbursement models were considered. The first, termed Model A, can be characterized as an incentive-based reimbursement approach used frequently in preferred provider organizations. In this approach, the consumer assumes financial responsibility for a 20 percent copayment if nonparticipating providers are used; if the preferred panel is used, the consumer does

Table 4-1 Example of Employee Choice of Health Benefits Coverage with PPO and EPO Options

	EPO	PPO	Traditional Insurance	IPA Model HMO
Monthly employee contribution for family contract	$0	$20	$20	$38
Deductible	None	None as long as participating providers are used	$250	None
Maximum out-of-pocket	$1,000	$3,000	$3,000	Does not apply
In-Hospital				
Room and Board	Same as PPO	100%	80%	100%
Surgery	Same as PPO	100%	80%–50%	100%
Lab and X-Ray	Same as PPO	100%	80%	100%
Physician	Same as PPO	100%	80%	100%
Outpatient				
Doctor's Office	Same as PPO	100%	80%	You pay $5/visit
Routine Physicals	Same as PPO	100%	Not Covered	
Eye and Ear Exams	Same as PPO	100%	Not Covered	You pay $5/visit
Eyeglasses and Hearing Aids	Same as PPO	100%	Not Covered	100% through age 17
Maternity	Same as PPO	Not Covered	Not Covered	Not Covered
Lab and X-Ray	Same as PPO	90%	80%	100%
Immunizations	Same as PPO	100%	80%	100%
Ambulatory Surgery	Same as PPO	100%	Not Covered	100%
Ambulance	Same as PPO	100%	100%	100%
Hospice	Same as PPO	90% if medically necessary	First $50, plus 80% of balance	100%, if medically necessary
Durable Equipment	Same as PPO	100%	100%	Not Covered

Table 4-1 continued

	EPO	PPO	Traditional Insurance	IPA Model HMO
Psychiatric Benefit	Same as PPO	90%	80%	80% of purchase of rental price
Inpatient	Same as PPO	75% for 30 days/year	50% for 30 days/year	Not covered unless part of another medical condition
Outpatient	Same as PPO	75% for 50 visits/year	50% up to $40 for 30 visits/year	$20/visit for 20 visits/contract
Substance Abuse (Alcohol and Drugs) Inpatient	Same as PPO	90% for 30 days/year at designated facilities	80% for employee; 50% for dependents for 30 days/year	100% for short-term detoxification treatment
Outpatient	Same as PPO	100%	50% up to $40 for 30 visits/year	Not Covered
Outpatient Prescription Drugs		You pay $3/prescription at participating pharmacies	80%	You pay $3/prescription at participating pharmacies

not pay a copayment. Model B can be characterized as a disincentive approach. The consumer pays a 20 percent copayment even when the preferred panel is used for services. If non-PPO providers are used, however, the copayment increases to 40 percent. Model C typifies the exclusive provider organization arrangement. In this model, services rendered by the exclusive panel require no copayment. When nonpanel providers deliver care, the consumer faces a 100 percent copayment.

Table 4-2 illustrates the three different reimbursement models and the financial impact on a consumer faced with a provider charge of $300. Trauner assumed, for the purpose of this example, that the preferred provider organization negotiated a $250 charge for the service (a $50 discount). A further assumption was that the prevailing rate in the community for the particular service was $280. This represented the usual, customary, and reasonable (UCR) payment for that service. Trauner also reviewed different copayment levels that might be in force when a nonpreferred provider was used. A copayment might be calculated as a percent of the usual, customary, and reasonable fee or it may be calculated on the basis of the charge negotiated by the preferred provider organization.

The impact on the consumer can be substantial. Under incentive-type reimbursement (Model A) a patient using a nonpreferred provider would be charged $300. If the patient's copayment level was based on the UCR, the patient would pay $56 of the UCR ($280); the insurance carrier would pay the remainder of the UCR. However, the patient would be liable for the difference between the UCR and the actual physician charge. This represents an additional $20. Total out-of-pocket payments for the patient in this situation would be $76. If the copayment level was based on a percent of the negotiated PPO charge ($250), the patient would be required to contribute $50 while the insurance carrier paid $200. Again, however, there is a difference between the original physician charge to the patient and the amount covered by the insurance program. The patient in this instance would not only be faced with a $50 copayment; an additional $50 would have to be paid directly to the physician by the patient because the total insurance payment (carrier payment plus copayment) would have equaled only $250. Total out-of-pocket payment by the patient in this situation would be $100.

A review of Table 4-2 indicates that the total out-of-pocket payments by a patient increase substantially under the Model B type of reimbursement in which financial disincentives are used to encourage use of the preferred panel. In the most financially burdensome situation, a patient using a nonpreferred provider and faced with a 40 percent copayment (of the PPO negotiated charge), would pay $150 of a $300 physician bill.

In the EPO reimbursement model, an individual using a nonpreferred provider would be responsible for 100 percent of the charge. Thus, a patient failing to use one of the preferred providers would be confronted with total out-of-pocket costs of $300 on a $300 bill.

Table 4-2 Out-of-Pocket Medical Costs under Various PPO Reimbursement Models

Model	Provider $ Charge[1]	Percent Copayment[2]	$ Copayment	$ Difference between Charge & Reimbursement	Total Out-of-Pocket $ Cost[3]	% Total Bill as Out-of-Pocket (as % of UCR)
Model A (Incentive)						
PPO	$250	None	0	0	0	0
Non-PPO	300	20% of UCR	56	20	76	25.3% (27.1)
Non-PPO	300	20% of PPO	50	50	100	33.3 (35.7)
Model B (Disincentive)						
PPO	250	20% of PPO	50	0	50	20.4 (17.9)
Non-PPO	300	40% of UCR	112	20	132	44.0 (47.1)
Non-PPO	300	40% of PPO	100	50	150	50.0 (53.6)
Model C (EPO)						
PPO	250	None	0	0	0	0
Non-PPO	300	100%	300	0	300	100.0

Notes:

1. PPO negotiated charge is $250 (PPO); prevailing rate in community is $280 (UCR); non-PPO provider charge is $300.

2. For PPO users, copayment is calculated using negotiated rate of $250; for non-PPO users, two rates are provided, one calculated using UCR rate of $280, and the other, using PPO rate of $250.

3. Total out-of-pocket costs equal copayment plus difference between physician charge and reimbursement rate.

Source: Joan B. Trauner, *Preferred Provider Organizations: The California Experiment* (San Francisco: University of California, August 1983).

One primary conclusion can be drawn from Table 4-2 in the above cursory analysis: consumer cost sharing increases measurably under the disincentive (Model B) and exclusive provider (Model C) reimbursement arrangements. This suggests that the financial disincentives associated with Model B and C reimbursement systems are of such magnitude that they would strongly encourage the ongoing use of preferred professionals and facilities.

The implications of this observation are particularly important for physicians and hospitals considering PPO participation. It would appear to be in the best interest of such providers to advocate that the PPOs with which they are associated encourage purchaser groups to employ Model B and Model C reimbursement approaches. These seem to offer the best opportunity for increasing patient volume and market share of providers participating in the preferred panel organization.

Services Selection

A third level (tier) of consumer incentives has been included in select preferred provider programs. This third level recognizes that economic incentives may be required to ensure that consumers receive care in the most appropriate, least costly setting even when a preferred provider is being used. These incentives encourage the consumer/patient to "do the right thing in the right setting."

To achieve this goal, a consumer is presented with differential payment levels which strongly encourage appropriate behavior. That is, the PPO (through associated purchasers) may pay fully (100 percent), as an example, for select surgical procedures performed on an ambulatory basis. Conversely, the same service received on an inpatient basis might be covered at only 50 percent of cost. In the first instance, the consumer is economically rewarded for efficient medical decision making. The consumer in the latter case faces a financial penalty for less prudent buying behavior. Exhibit 4-1 identifies 44 elective surgical procedures that one purchaser required to be done in an outpatient setting in order for employees to have the costs of care covered at 100 percent.

The concept of providing disincentives for inappropriate consumer behavior can be extended to many areas other than ambulatory surgery. The concept of differential payment (e.g., 100 percent payment for "correct behavior," 50 percent for "inappropriate behavior") can be used to stimulate consumer cost consciousness in other situations:

- Second surgical opinions: patients that do not acquire second (or third) opinions on select elective surgical procedures must pay 50 percent of the cost of such treatment (see Exhibit 4-2).
- Preadmission certification and concurrent length of stay review: patients who disregard preadmission certification or length of stay determinations become liable for 50 percent of the cost of treatment.

Exhibit 4-1 Mandatory Outpatient Surgical Procedures

- Adenoidectomy
- Antral puncture
- Antrotomy
- Biopsy of: cervix
  breast
  muscle
- Cast change
- Cervical node biopsy
- Circumcision (adult)
- Cryotherapy
  e.g. skin, verruca
- Cystoscopy
- Dermabrasion
- Dilation of lacrimal duct
- Dilation and curettage of uterus
- Endoscopic exam
  e.g. arthroscopy
  esophagoscopy
  sigmoidoscopy
- Examination under anesthesia
  (pelvic exam)

- Excision of: Non-malignant
  e.g. Lipoma
  Neoplasm
  Nevi
  Papillomas
  Polyps
  Sebaceous cysts
  Warts
- Fractures
- Hymenotomy
- Hysterosalpingogram
- Hernia
- Incision and drainage cyst, abscess
- Incision and removal of foreign body, subcutaneous tissue, simple
- Lacerations
- Manipulations of joints
- Marsupialization of Bartholin cyst
- Meatotomy
- Myringotomy w/ or w/o tubes

- Operations on canthus
- Operations on external ear
- Otoplasty
- Paracentesis
- Probing of lacrimal duct
- Rectal polypectomy
- Removal of calculus and drainage of bladder w/o incision
- Removal of nail, nailbed, or nailfold
- Scar plasty
- Skin graft (minor)
- Sterilization (f) by laparoscopy including by mini-laparoscopy
- Tonsillectomy
- Tonsillectomy w/ adenoidectomy
- Tenotomy, hand or foot
- Tranfusion of blood
- Vasectomy
- Z-plasty for relaxation of scar or with contracture

- Medical Services Advisory Program: patients failing to review recommended (elective) hospital treatment with designated medical service advisory personnel assume responsibility for 50 percent of the cost care. (The medical advisory concept is discussed below.)

Preadmission testing and weekend admissions represent additional situations in which differential payment can be used to produce substantial economic incentives.

PPOs do not seem to have aggressively and widely applied the concept of differential payments. This has been so in large part because (1) the decision to implement differential payment is a function of individual purchasers who are linked to the PPO, not the PPO itself, and (2) PPOs have generally required providers to assume responsibility for using cost-efficient settings like ambulatory surgery.

Exhibit 4-2 Surgical Procedures for Which Second Opinions Are Often Strongly Encouraged

● Bunionectomy	● Mastectomy and other operations of breast
● Cholecystectomy	● Myringotomy with or without tubes
● Coronary bypass surgery	● Prostatectomy
● Septal reconstruction	● Removal of cataract
● Hernia repair	● Tonsillectomy and/or adenoidectomy
● Hysterectomy	● Varicose vein excision and ligation
● Knee surgery	● Laminectomy

INFORMING CONSUMERS

The multitiered system of incentives/disincentives represents the most fundamental way to influence consumer purchasing behavior. Such systems of incentives are the tools used most frequently to shape consumer behavior. Information-based mechanisms can also be used to achieve similar purposes. These include (1) predetermination of benefits and (2) medical services advisory programs.

Predetermination of Benefits (POB)

The national movement to increase employee participation in the payment of rendered medical care provides PPOs with the opportunity to identify for consumers the financial implications of their purchasing decisions. Predetermination of Benefits (POB) is a process that directly provides consumers with cost-related information. Most typically, this is performed when inpatient services or high-cost ambulatory services are necessary.

The core of the POB process is the POB form, shown in Exhibit 4-3. Information on a patient's diagnoses, procedures to be performed or services to be rendered, and the estimated cost of treatment are identified by the patient's physician. With such data in hand, a PPO is in a position to inform a patient about the amount to be covered by the purchaser and, conversely, the estimated amount for which the patient becomes responsible. Some companies, like Georgia's West Point Pepperell, use the POB process without PPO application.

The value of the POB process is that it offers a patient prospective information on the cost of care; when large or excessive out-of-pocket costs appear likely, the patient still has an opportunity to defer his or her decision about those physicians and hospitals that might ultimately be used. Preferred provider arrangements can expect to be viewed favorably when such purchasing decisions are made by consumers.

Exhibit 4-3 Predetermination of Benefits Estimation Inquiry

WestPoint Pepperell
GROUP HEALTH AND DISABILITY PLAN

PREDETERMINATION OF BENEFITS ESTIMATION INQUIRY

The purpose of this inquiry is to provide the employee with information that will help him plan financially for non-emergency medical care. It is optional and is available at the employee's request.

_____PART A – TO BE COMPLETED BY EMPLOYEE_____

Physician _____   Date _____

Address _____

_____   Physician's

_____   Phone No.   _____

Employee_____SSN_____   Where
Employed_____

Dependent _____Relation _____   Effective Date
of Coverage _____

Place of Service:

☐ Hospital   ☐ IP   ☐ OP   Name _____

☐ Free Standing Ambulatory   City _____
   Surgical Clinic

☐ Physician's Office   State_____

_____PART B – TO BE COMPLETED BY PHYSICIAN_____

Diagnosis. (The reason the treatment is necessary.)   ICD-9 Diagnosis Code

_____   _____

_____   _____

_____   _____

_____   _____

Description of the anticipated service.   CPT-4   Estimated Cost
(Please identify any separate charges.)   Procedure Code   of Service

_____   _____   _____

_____   _____   _____

_____   _____   _____

_____   _____   _____

THIS IS NOT A CLAIM FORM

Exhibit 4-3 continued

_____PART C - TO BE COMPLETED IN THE GROUP INSURANCE CLAIMS OFFICE_____

Identified CPT-4 Procedure Code	Estimated Cost of Service From Supplier	Estimated Covered Expense*	Estimated Non-Covered Expense*	Explanation Non-Covered Expense
_____	_____	_____	_____	_____
_____	_____	_____	_____	_____
_____	_____	_____	_____	_____
_____	_____	_____	_____	_____
_____	_____	_____	_____	_____

If an Assistant Surgeon's fee is covered, the fee considered will be 20% of the Primary Surgeon's reasonable and customary fee.

PLEASE ATTACH A COPY OF THIS FORM TO THE CLAIM WHEN IT IS FILED

Comments _____

_____

_____

_____

_____

_____

_____

EXPLANATION OF NON-COVERED EXPENSE:

Code A: The estimated charge is higher than the reasonable and customary benefit indicated for this geographic region.

Code B: The condition is identified as pre-existing – coverage is not in effect.

Code C: The identified service is not covered by the Plan.

Code D: More information is needed. (See Comments)

*These figures are only an estimation and are based only on the services described in this inquiry.

"Covered Expense" means the amount that would be **considered** covered by the WestPoint Pepperell Group Health and Disability Plan **on the date of the inquiry response**. "Covered Expenses" are further defined on pages 16 and 17 of the Group Health and Disability Plan, Summary Plan Description.

Copy to:

☐ Employee   ☐ Personnel Department   Response Date _____

☐ Physician   ☐ File   Signature _____

WP-17773-H

Source: Health Care Benefits Department, West Point Pepperell, Group Health and Benefits Plan, West Point, Georgia.

The Medical Services Advisory Program

A more personalized refinement of the POB process is the Medical Services Advisory Program (MSAP). Medical Services Advisory Programs, to date, have been operational only at corporate (but not PPO) levels. Zenith Corporation in Chicago and Pratt Whitney in Florida provide examples of purchasers that have instituted MSAPs. The ability of these programs to influence patient cost consciousness and, consequently, the use of a preferred panel of providers, strongly suggests that PPOs will increasingly adopt this innovation in the future.

The basic purpose of an MSAP is to advise an employee/patient who requires costly outpatient or inpatient services about the following:

- The cost of care the patient will assume based on provider selection and benefits coverage
- Alternatives the patient may wish to consider if inpatient care has been recommended: ambulatory options, preadmission testing, appropriate lower-cost facilities, etc.
- The expected length of stay and the extent to which additional nonapproved days will be covered

The obvious advantage of an MSAP over POB is that it allows personal contact (nurse, medical director) as the tool for exploring cost-controlling options, even within the context of a preferred provider program.[2]

Zenith Radio Corporation's program provides insight into the type of information-based initiatives PPOs are likely to incorporate in the future.[3] Zenith initiated a series of cost-containment changes, in conjunction with its claims administrator, Blue Cross/Blue Shield of Illinois, in 1981. This series of changes was initially based on an analysis of claims data that highlighted average length of stay, diagnosis, and institutional cost comparisons. This initial analysis found that lengthy hospital stays were a principal problem. In addition to other benefit changes, Zenith added a medical services adviser to its medical department in 1983. The adviser has a medical background and utilization review experience as well as a knowledge about insurance benefits. Employees are required to inform the adviser about the medical procedures recommended by a physician, the hospital at which services are scheduled to be provided, diagnosis, anticipated length of stay, and day of week of admission. The adviser provides suggestions about less costly settings for care when applicable, the appropriateness of the length of stay, and related matters. It has been estimated that the program will save as much as 10 percent. Further, initial physician response to the program has been favorable. Informal reports suggest that area physicians have shown a willingness to cooperate when presented with requests for ambulatory, rather than inpatient, services, or for the use of a less costly hospital when uncomplicated conditions are being treated.

The medical services advisory concept is not a panacea for correcting inappropriate consumer behavior. MSAP personnel would naturally need to possess significant amounts of information on purchaser insurance/medical benefit programs and coverage levels. In a setting involving many purchasers with widely divergent coverage levels, the goal of accurately advising each PPO consumer might prove unattainable. An additional problem—consumer nonparticipation— might also exist. In order to approach effectiveness, consumers must use the MSAP regularly. The use of economic incentives/disincentives, or a mandatory requirement that consumers contact the MSAP when hospitalization has been recommended, may be necessary.

CONCLUDING PERSPECTIVE

The traditional notion that the mere addition of copayments, coinsurance, and deductibles can uniformly produce consumer cost consciousness is being replaced by more refined incentive/disincentive systems. Preferred provider programs have made wide use of economic incentives to influence provider choice, yet these incentives do not necessarily guarantee appropriate service utilization. Service-specific incentives, based on differential payment, and consumer information programs can be expected to be gradually adopted by PPO purchasers and programs.

NOTES

1. Joan B. Trauner, *Preferred Provider Organizations: The California Experiment* (San Francisco: University of California, August 1983), 12–19.

2. P. Torrens, "The Company Doctor Is In," *Health Cost Management* 1, no. 2 (November 1983): 7–9.

3. S.J. Drury, "Zenith Uses Claims Data To Cut Health Costs," *Business Insurance* (May 23, 1983): 3+.

Chapter 5

Cost Efficiency and the Medical Provider

The national interest in preferred provider organizations has been strongly influenced by the perceived ability of these delivery systems to restrain health costs and utilization. The establishment of cost-containing devices has not been the result of the acceptance of financial risk as is the case with health maintenance organizations. Rather, PPOs illustrate a definite response to the contemporary health marketplace in which, increasingly, resources are being shifted away from open-ended financing/delivery systems toward those that demonstrate both an interest in, and ability to, control health costs. This observation partially explains the ability of early PPO-like arrangements to operate, at least initially, by offering only discounted services. The absence of financial risk allowed this behavior; it was not until purchasers began to demand stronger controls that utilization review and other cost-control instruments were employed.

Cost efficiency is frequently discussed only in terms of discounts and utilization restraints. Yet innovative, visionary organizations recognize that these two mechanisms are not the universe of cost control and that those who mistakenly assume this will face stiff competition in the future from more aggressive and creative challengers. In addition to discounts and utilization review, other tools for PPO cost efficiency are[1]

1. The conscious selection of efficient physicians and hospitals
2. Financial arrangements that produce economic rewards for efficient provider behavior, particularly that of physicians
3. Information feedback systems that constantly and quantitatively illustrate to physicians their practice efficiency relative to other practitioners.

The purpose of each tool is to alter physician and hospital behavior in ways that enhance efficiency and cost containment.

SELECTING EFFICIENT PROVIDERS

The selection of efficient hospitals and physicians is one of the most difficult, though crucial, tasks a PPO undertakes. The sizable number of providers to be screened complicates the selection process. Although hospitals would seem to be the logical and primary focus of the selection process, they are not. They are secondary to the identification and selection of those professionals who are the force that determines the efficiency or inefficiency of a preferred arrangement: the physicians.

Selecting Physicians

The selection of efficient physicians is, in its most fundamental form, a function of three tasks:

1. Ensuring that applicant physicians provide qualitatively adequate services
2. Determining that any individual physician's hospital practice pattern results in very reasonable average stays and total charges per patient
3. Determining that physicians use inpatient resources most judiciously.

Methodologies for addressing these three matters are, in most instances, less than fully developed. Data on quality matters and practice patterns are rarely available and are typically subjective in nature. Even in instances when subjective qualitative assessment may be possible, perhaps through a hospital quality assurance director, and in situations where data on the charges and patient lengths of stay are available, a PPO still may not have access to the third essential item of information: the frequency with which a physician admits patients for unnecessary inpatient services. Indeed, inefficient practitioners may appear unusually efficient when only length of stay and charges are considered since nonacute patients can be discharged more quickly than those truly requiring hospitalization.

The difficulty in selecting efficient providers has resulted, generally, in the application of PPO physician participation criteria that do not explicitly consider practice efficiency. The criteria, rather, require acceptable standing within quality of care parameters, articulated by the applicable medical staff and associations like state medical societies. Further, physicians most often agree contractually to the utilization review process in which quality and efficiency are monitored. Last, PPO contracts stipulate the reasons for which physician participation may be terminated.

It is important to note that the majority of preferred arrangements operate in the above fashion. Stringent efficiency criteria are being used once a practitioner has been accepted into the PPO environment, not as a prerequisite for participation. There exist, however, a limited number of examples in which efficiency criteria are being prospectively applied.

Pratt-Whitney Aircraft has used subjective qualitative judgment as an approach to identifying physicians who are subsequently recommended to employees. This represents an informal type of PPO. In the late '70s, Pratt-Whitney's medical director was confronted by a number of employees who were disturbed by physician bills that exceeded the UCR amount paid by the company's insurer; the employees were financially responsible for the portion of the charges not covered by the insurance plan.

In an effort to alter this situation, the medical director contacted local physicians he knew personally and/or in whom he had professional confidence. These physicians agreed to accept the UCR payment as payment in full.

The physician selection approach used by Pratt-Whitney emphasized collegial and peer respect. Panel physicians were invited to participate in the informal panel by a colleague (the medical director) who had subjectively determined that the quality and cost of their services were of an acceptable nature.

Today, the program boasts a panel of about 150 physicians who agree to care for Pratt-Whitney employees. The only incentive these employees have to request services from panel members is the possibility that they may be charged for physician costs above those covered by the insurance plan if nonpanel physicians are used.

Independence Medical Systems, an investor-owned PPO developing in Clearwater, Florida, has applied a similar technique for selecting physician participants. One of the investors is a practicing physician who initially identified a small number of medical colleagues (about 60) considered to be providers of high-quality, cost-efficient care. As the PPO develops, this group of hand-picked practitioners will establish criteria for future physician involvement.

The system used by the Greater Baltimore PPO is perhaps the best example of a process in which extensive data exists for provider selection. The Maryland Health Care Services Cost Review Commission continuously collects physician-specific information, by diagnostic group, on the practice efficiency of individual providers. This information is publicly available and has been used extensively by the Greater Baltimore PPO. Tables 5-1 and 5-2 illustrate the format used for the presentation of physician-specific information.

The process used by the Baltimore Preferred Provider Organization is direct and straightforward. In the early stages of development (during 1983) the PPO identified the primary hospitals with which it wished to affiliate. Once these facilities had been identified, respected senior physicians on the staffs of each facility were asked to subjectively delineate those practitioners who, based on their knowledge, exhibited high-quality and cost-efficient practice styles. The physicians who undertook this initial screening process were typically physicians with substantial utilization review and quality assessment experience at the re-

Table 5-1 Physician Efficiency Indicators as Measured by Days Above Average (DAA) and Percent Above Average (PAA)

Maryland
Health Services Cost Review Commission
Physician Report Part 1
Data Period = 1980 Year

Hospital: XXXX

Physician No.	Patient Days	Expected Number of Days	Days Above Ave.	% Above Ave.
000123	663	352.04	310.96	88.33
000238	1719	1415.15	303.85	21.47
000226	1205	978.63	226.37	23.13
000236	978	792.45	185.55	23.42
000205	819	672.85	146.15	21.72
800000	871	757.86	113.14	14.93
000219	1112	1004.62	107.38	10.69
600000	758	701.45	56.55	8.06

Source: Alvin D. Ankrum, *Analyzing Hospital Utilization and Efficiency* (Baltimore, Md.: Baltimore City Professional Standards Review Organization, February 1981).

spective hospitals and as a result were in a position to evaluate the quality and efficiency of possible candidates.

The identification of physicians provided the foundation for considering objective, statistical information collected by the Maryland Health Services Cost Review Commission. The principal efficiency statistics examined were Charges Above Average (CAA) and Days Above Average (DAA). As illustrated in Table 5-1, diagnosis-specific information, based on Diagnostically Related Groups (DRGs), compares a physician's patients' average length of stay with an area average. Days above this average represent the DAA statistic. The diagnostically specific DAA information, when aggregated, provides an associated statistic, the percent above average. Again, this is illustrated in Table 5-1. The table shows that, for the physicians compared, the range in the percent of days above average has a low of about 8 percent and a high of over 88 percent.

The Greater Baltimore Preferred Provider Organization (GBPPO) combined the subjective and objective assessments to produce a listing of those physicians the organization wished to have participate.

There are two points of interest to note with respect to this particular preferred provider organization. First, the PPO's marketing program is designed largely around the selection process. That is, the GBPPO gives substantial visibility to its qualitative and cost-efficiency characteristics. The efficiency of participating

Table 5-2 DRG Specific Days Above Average for an Individual Physician

Maryland
Health Services Cost Review Commission
Physician Report Part 2
Date Period = 1980 Year

Hospital: XXXX
Physician No. 000XXX*

DRG	Pts.	Ave. LOS	Area Ave.	Days Over Ave.	DRG Titles
79	1	16.00	9.73	6.27	Metabolic DIS of Gout, Globulinopathy, Xanthomatosis W-DX2
299	1	11.00	5.03	5.97	DIS of bone & cartilage w excision semilunar cart, repair Oth joint
302	2	8.00	5.53	4.94	Bunion, Synovitis, Bursitis, Tenosynovitis, Scoliosis, Deform Foot wo oper
307	2	8.50	7.56	1.88	Oth DIS of Musculoskeletal Syst (major) w excsn. repair (SML JNT, bone)
310	1	19.00	6.15	12.85	Cong Anomaly (heart, kidney, Oth major) wo oper
312	5	7.20	4.67	12.65	Cong Anom of heart (valve, unspec) w heart catheterization
313	6	7.33	6.13	7.22	Cong Anom (palate, lip, hip, Oth extr) w repair (lip, palate). Arthrodesis
315	1	9.00	5.37	3.63	ASD, TOF, PDA, COA, Hypospadia w catheterization, repair urethra
316	5	20.00	14.55	27.25	ASD, TOF, PDA, COA w oper on valve, septum, shunt
380	26	13.92	5.69	214.06	Followup (CA), SURG-MED after care (Colostomy, Orthop, Oth) wo oper
382	7	4.71	2.68	14.24	Special admission w cystoscopy, removal of fix device (internal)
TOTAL	57	11.63		310.96	

*Concealed for display purposes only.

Source: Alvin D. Ankrum, *Analyzing Hospital Utilization and Efficiency* (Baltimore, Md.: Baltimore City Professional Standards Review Organization, February 1981).

physicians and the inability of organizations to negotiate hospital discounts in Maryland because of legislated hospital rate control has resulted in a preferred provider organization that offers neither physician nor hospital discounts to subscribing purchasers. The second noteworthy point is that the selection process has had an apparently beneficial impact on those physicians not involved in the organization. Anecdotal reports indicate that physicians not invited to participate have inquired as to the reasons for their exclusion. PPO officials have pointed out to them that their practice characteristics as reported by the Maryland Health Services Cost Review Commission precluded participation. Some physicians have been unaware of the existence of the data. Others have asked about the possibility of future involvement if practice statistics improve. The Greater Baltimore PPO has informally indicated to physicians that improvements in practice characteristics may open the door to future PPO association.

The Physicians' Alliance for Medical Excellence is located in Lexington, Kentucky. It is an organization established by physicians. The Physicians' Alliance has several stated participation criteria including board certification or eligibility, participation in general peer review and quality assurance activities, and a genuine interest in health promotion and patient education. In addition, though, participation criteria include the submission of Blue Cross/Blue Shield reports comparing an individual physician's inpatient hospital cost record with that of peers. The peer group is defined as physicians in Kentucky of the same specialty practicing at hospitals of a similar size. Physicians are compared and ranked within their peer group on several variables: average total bill, average length of stay, laboratory charges, medication charges, and x-ray charges. The data used by the Alliance ranks a physician with the number 1 if the physician has the highest cost within his or her peer group. Rankings of high numbers indicate increasing cost efficiency as determined by these particular reports. Based on 1982 Blue Cross/Blue Shield of Kentucky data, Physicians' Alliance members exhibited total hospital costs per case that were 15 percent less than peer averages; average lengths of stay were 11 percent less. Table 5-3 contains an example of the Blue Cross/Blue Shield reports used by the Physicians' Alliance.

A similar physician selection system is used by the Physicians' Alliance of Roanoke (Virginia). This organization was assisted in its development by staff of the Lexington group.

The Mid-America Health Network is a Kansas City, Missouri-based preferred provider organization using a selection process similar to that employed by Lexington's Physicians' Alliance. The Mid-America Health Network is a for-profit corporation established by several inpatient facilities in the Kansas City area. Program officials began the operational phase in May 1984. The Network is linked contractually with Mid-America Medical Affiliates, the physician component of the preferred provider arrangement. Participation criteria for Mid-

Table 5-3 Practice Data Submitted by Physicians Prior to Acceptance into the Physicians' Alliance for Medical Excellence

Physician: XXXXX
Specialty: Gastroenterology
Hospital: 141
Period: January 1982–December 1982

Ancillary Area	Total* Cases	Ranking within** Peer Group	Peer Average	Individual Average
Laboratory	77	11 of 18	$228.82	$189.25
Medication	73	4 of 18	$285.27	$328.79
X-Ray	66	10 of 18	$253.28	$250.72
Total Bill	77	13 of 18	$2019.42	$1854.76
Average Length of Stay	77	10 of 18	6.90 Days	6.68 Days

*Total cases include all regular Blue Cross inpatient claims paid during the period, at the hospital listed, on which the physician is designated as the admitting physician. If the patient is later referred to the services of another physician, the entire case remains on the admitting physician's summary.

**The peer group consists of physicians having the same specialty and practicing at facilities of the same general size. The ranking within peer group is in descending order. For example: a ranking of #1 represents the highest average cost within the peer group.

Source: Physicians' Alliance for Medical Excellence, Lexington, Kentucky (personal communication).

America Affiliates require that applying physicians sign a release allowing the acquisition of PSRO data. The PSRO information is diagnosis specific and computes differences between an individual physician's patients' length of stay and defined averages.

Physician Selection Processes and the Future

It can be anticipated that the processes used for selecting physicians or allowing their participation will become more vigorous as competition between preferred provider organizations heightens. Other highly competitive health delivery systems like U.S. Health Care Systems, Inc., have employed more aggressive approaches. Although it is an IPA model HMO, it offers a glimpse of the physician selection processes of the future.[2]

Prior to 1981, U.S. Health Care Systems, Inc. (USHCSI), operated as a nonprofit, community-based organization known as The Health Maintenance Organization of Pennsylvania (HMO/PA). USHCSI was established in September 1981. This new corporate entity was investor owned and assumed virtually all the assets, liabilities, and ongoing operations of HMO/PA. The name of the predecessor organization was maintained for business purposes. The nonprofit predecessor was also used and continues to be used as a private foundation for education and community services.

The financial risk assumed by this IPA model health maintenance organization, as well as its relatively new investor-owned status, have required that the organization operate an aggressive physician selection program. The selection process begins with a formal written application detailing information on a physician's qualifications, office practice, arrangements for around-the-clock coverage, patient load, etc. In addition, physicians are required to submit at least four letters of recommendation. One of these letters must come from a physician who is currently a member of the IPA. Following the submission of the application and recommendations, an interview with one of the organization's medical directors is arranged and site visits are conducted. The applicant is asked to provide medical charts for review by the director. The site visits and the review of medical charts for each individual applicant place a strong emphasis on both quality and cost efficiency.

Recommendations of the director, as well as application forms, are eventually submitted to an executive committee, which makes a final determination about a physician's participation. But physician participation is not absolute. That is, acceptance into the organization is based initially on a two-year provisional period. During the provisional period, the physician's practice is reviewed and data is collected and discussed further with appropriate committees and individuals within the IPA. If the general practice standards of the IPA are maintained during the provision period, the physician is eventually accepted as an active member. It is estimated that between 15 and 20 percent of all applicants are denied the initial provisional status.

The office site visit and the review of medical charts conducted by United States Health Care Systems, Inc., have important implications for the PPO movement as well as other types of alternative delivery systems. At the beginning of this discussion on physician selection procedures, it was noted that three tasks must be satisfactorily completed. Quality must be assured, average length of stay and total charges must be appropriate, and the rate of admissions should be judicious. There do not appear to be any preferred provider organizations that currently have access to information on admission rates and the level of inappropriate admissions. The site visits and chart reviews conducted by U.S. Health Care Systems, Inc., however, allow for the possibility of such rates to be established or subjectively noted.

The Non Acute Profile (NAP) is one technical tool that preferred provider organizations may turn to in an effort to accurately determine the extent of inappropriate or unnecessary hospitalization.[3] The Non Acute Profile, as its name suggests, applies specific criteria to hospitalizations in order to determine patterns of non acute hospital admissions and/or services. The NAP was developed by the Delmarva Foundation for Medical Care in Easton, Maryland, and is based on criteria developed by Paul M. Gertman, M.D., as part of his research on the Appropriateness Evaluation Protocol. The Gertman approach is formulated on a criteria set based on objectively observable items that are easily obtained from hospital records. Delmarva's Non Acute Profile is obtained by applying the criteria to documented information contained in hospital medical records. If specific services or conditions are not present on the day being studied, the day is described as a non acute day of hospitalization. The criteria can be applied uniformly and, largely, inflexibly. This produces an objective comparison of non acute use rates by physicians (and hospitals).

Exhibit 5-1 illustrates an NAP for an individual physician performed by the Delmarva Foundation for Medical Care. The profile is for a specific physician and the percent of total days found to be non acute for the individual physician is compared with that of physicians of a similar specialty. The NAP methodology classifies non acute days according to the principal reasons for the non acute determination. Frequent reasons include delays in ordering patient discharge, non acute admission, early admission, delays in locating lower levels of care (such as nursing care), patient/family factors, delays in ancillary or consulting services, and delays in the ordering of ancillary or consulting services. Exhibit 5-1 illustrates that for the physician being studied, non acute days were recorded at a rate twice that of the physician's peers. The particular physician reported a non acute percentage of 50 percent of all days as non acute, while the peer group average was approximately 26 percent. An examination of the reasons for the physician's non acute record illustrates that the physician in question grossly

Exhibit 5-1 Example of Physician Specific Non Acute Profile, Delmarva
Foundation for Medical Care

```
Physician Name: XXXXXXXXXXXXX
Time Period: Oct. 1980–Sept. 1981
Specialty: Orthopedics

                    Peer Physicians,
     Physician      Orthopedics
       50%            25.7%        Total Non Acute Percent in Sample
       19%             6.1%        Delay in Ordering Discharge
       12%             6.4%        Non Acute Admission
        8%             2.1%        Early Admission
       12%             7.3%        Waiting for Lower Level of Care
        0%             2.1%        Patient/Family Factors
        0%             1.5%        Delay in Ordering Ancillary/Consult
        0%             0%          Ancillary/Consult Delay

         The following display represents your total non acute percentages for a
         baseline period and for recent months.
                   July 80–Mar. 81        Apr. 81–Sep. 81
                       47%                     62%

Patients with Non Acute Days:
(Only patients reviewed during the most recent three months are listed. Complete lists for the
most recent year are available on request.)

     Record #       Admission Date    Reason for Non Acute Day(s)
     220-18-3          6-9-81          Waiting for Lower Level of Care
     564-44-5          8-4-81          Delay in Ordering Discharge
     218-20-6          7-18-81         Early Admission & Delay in Ordering Discharge
     220-09-1          9-1-81          Delay in Ordering Discharge

     Note: Non acute profiles merely display data variations as do length of stay variation profiles.
     Physician peer review is required to determine whether a non acute day is inappropriate.
```

exceeded peer group averages for (1) delays in ordering patient discharges,
(2) non acute admissions, and (3) early admissions.

It is important to recognize that the NAP utilized by the Delmarva Foundation
for Medical Care does not define whether the non acute day is inappropriate.
Rather, physician peer review is required to examine non acute days in greater
detail in order to determine whether such days are truly inappropriate.

The NAP has several important and beneficial characteristics which suggest
that this method may be used more frequently in the future to prospectively
identify physicians most appropriate for involvement in PPOs. The NAP methodology can be employed on a sample basis, using a 10 or 20 percent sample
of the admissions generated by a particular physician. Further, the nature of the

profile is such that it accounts for the severity and diagnostic condition of patients. These two important characteristics help to make the NAP a potentially powerful addition to the physician selection process. One can easily envision a physician application process that would involve the following:

1. A physician interested in participating in the preferred provider organization would submit an application for participation. Part of that application would require that the physician allow a sample of his or her discharges to be examined using the NAP methodology.
2. The NAP would be conducted.
3. The results of the profile would be compared with previously defined limits on the percent of non acute days that are acceptable for any specialty and the percent of non acute days attributable to non acute admissions. (Mean non acute day percentages for various specialties are presented in Table 5-4.)

The NAP, then, could directly facilitate the examination of admission practice patterns discussed above. Physicians whose percent of non acute days resulting from non acute admissions exceeded previously defined limits could, in general, be prohibited from PPO involvement.

Table 5-4 Delmarva Foundation for Medical Care Non Acute Profile Variation: By Specialty

Specialty	Mean Non Acute Percent	Lowest Percent	Highest Percent
Neurology	26.4%	12%	52%
Orthopedics	25.1%	0%	39%
Thoracic Surgery	21.1%	12%	33%
General Surgery	17.5%	0%	44%
General Practice	16.9%	0%	67%
Otolaryngology	16.9%	0%	44%
Cardiology	16.5%	0%	39%
Internal Medicine	15.1%	0%	42%
Gastroenterology	14.9%	4%	58%
Obstetrics/Gynecology	11.6%	0%	22%
Urology	9.7%	0%	21%
Psychiatry	8.6%	0%	15%
Ophthalmology	2.7%	0%	10%
Oral Surgery	0.0%	0%	0%
TOTAL	15.7%	0%	67%

The cost of employing the NAP as a screening device is substantial but not prohibitive.[4] The Delmarva Foundation prefers to examine at least 20 patient charts before an NAP is prepared for any given physician. The cost is $15, or $300 per physician for a sample of 20 charts. A PPO screening 400 physicians would face NAP screening fees of $120,000, equal to the cost of less than 50 average hospital admissions.

Selecting Hospitals

The determination of hospital efficiency, and the eventual involvement of efficient facilities in preferred provider organizations, is, like physician selection, a complex task that has not been vigorously undertaken by many organizations. The infrequency with which hospital efficiency has been assessed can be explained by two factors. First, a large number of existing and developmental preferred provider organizations have been set up by individual or groups of hospitals. Common sense suggests that such facilities have little interest in quantifying what they already know. Second, the efficiency level of an individual hospital may be only of marginal interest to a preferred provider organization if the facility is capable of providing the PPO with substantial discounts from billed charges, or is willing to enter into at-risk financial arrangements. Supporters of this perspective would suggest that the imposition of strong utilization controls by the preferred provider organization, and the acquisition of substantial discounts, allow for a large margin of inefficiency before the PPO is adversely affected. Hopefully, such views are in a decisive minority; gross inefficiencies avoided by one purchaser can be and historically have been easily shifted to those purchasers of less influence.

The fundamental system used for the selection of hospitals is based on analysis of average cost per day or admission. In any community these costs may vary by as much as 200 percent. Community Hospital A may charge, on the average, $3,000 for a normal delivery; Hospital B, two blocks away, may necessarily charge $6,000 for the same service in order to support other more intensive services and the teaching/research programs it offers. In such environments, the job of the preferred provider organization is to select and eventually contract with those institutions (1) providing high-quality, low-cost care and (2) exhibiting acceptable community reputations and adequate geographic distribution.

Table 5-5 offers a comparison of ratios of the 1981 average daily charges for hospitals in the Clearwater, Florida, area. This information was used by Independence Medical Systems of Clearwater to identify lower-cost, high-quality facilities and also as a basis for eventual contract negotiation. The table shows that the lowest-cost hospital in the area is 50 percent less costly per day than the average of all hospitals. Further, the most expensive facility reports daily costs that are twice that of the lowest-cost institution.

Table 5-5 Comparison Ratios of 1981 Average Daily Charge,* Pinellas County, Florida

Hospital	Mean	Ratios Based on Lowest Price	Mean	Ratios Based on 2nd Lowest Price
#1	$266.15	1.00		.80
#2		1.25		1.00
#3		1.27		1.02
#4		1.32		1.06
#5		1.39		1.11
#6		1.43		1.15
#7		1.47		1.18
#8		1.48		1.19
#9		1.50		1.20
#10	$400.62	1.53		1.22
			$409.57	
#11		1.57		1.26
#12		1.60		1.28
#13		1.66		1.33
#14		1.68		1.34
#15		1.19		1.53
#16	$539.50	2.03		1.62

*Average gross daily charges (before contractual allowances) to all patients—1981. Average daily charges to commercial insurance patients tend to be 15–20% lower than the average charge to all patients.

Source: Independence Medical Systems, Clearwater, Florida (personal communication).

The executives of Independence Medical Systems, as well as health professionals in general, recognize that average daily charges or average charge per admission can be influenced by many factors. The severity level of patients seen by individual facilities and the mix of diagnostic conditions treated are two factors that largely determine the cost of care rendered. In the absence of diagnosis-specific information or severity of illness data, subjective assessment by medical professionals is the tool employed most frequently by preferred provider organizations to consider the influence of these factors. Independence Medical Systems, for example, uses the expertise of a physician investor to assist with such value judgments.

The recent publication of a hospital-specific Medicare Case-Mix Index may offer preferred provider organizations a new dimension in selecting cost-efficient institutions.[5] The Medicare Case-Mix Index (CMI) is a ratio that compares an individual hospital's expected average cost for the types of Medicare cases it treats with the national Medicare average cost per case. The Index is expressed relative to a national average index of 1.0. A hospital with an index of 1.5 is expected to have costs per case that are one and one-half times the national average. As of September 1983, the Index ranged from a low of .50 to an approximate high of 1.65. Reliability and validity studies published by the Health Care Financing Administration have concluded that the CMI is a significant factor in explaining hospital costs. The studies by the Health Care Financing Administration have concluded that hospitals, for example, having a 10 percent higher CMI should have a cost per case that is also 10 percent higher than the average.[6] This increased cost reflects the more complex case mix experienced by such institutions.

The Medicare Case-Mix Index cannot be used as an absolute indicator of hospital efficiency. It does, however, provide a very rough indicator not previously available for all hospitals. In attempting to assess, in a very general manner, the efficiency of individual institutions, the following process has been employed:[7]

1. The average charge per case for Medicare patients would be obtained by the PPO from published or internal sources.
2. The average charge per case for all patients would be used in those instances when Medicare data is unavailable. This procedure is not necessarily recommended. If it is used, however, it should be used for all institutions. That is, the average charge per case for all institutions should be either for total patients or for the Medicare population; it should not be a mixture of the two.
3. The average charge per case is divided by the CMI, resulting in a mathematical adjustment of the average charge per case, which, in a very gross sense, reflects case mix.

The process of dividing the average charge by the CMI has two results. When the CMI is less than 1 (indicating a less complex case mix), the average charge per case will increase. Conversely, a CMI greater than 1.0 will reduce the average charge per case. The CMI-adjusted cost per case can then be ranked and considered to be a rough indicator of hospital efficiency. Table 5-6 provides an example of how this might be performed. If one were to consider only the actual charge per case contained in Table 5-6, one would immediately conclude that hospitals A and B were the most efficient. Case-mix adjustment produces a very interesting result, however. Hospital A becomes the most inefficient institution based on this method and its assumptions. Hospital B presents very respectable CMI-adjusted costs per case and is ranked as one of the more efficient institutions.

Likewise, hospitals, E, F, and G would appear to be overly costly, and potentially inefficient, based on the reported average cost per case. When the cost per case is adjusted by the Medicare Case-Mix Index, hospitals F and G

Table 5-6 Estimating Hospital Efficiency Through the Use of the Medicare Case-Mix Index: An Illustration

Hospital	CMI	Average Charge Per Case	CMI Adjusted Charge Per Case	Efficiency Rank
A	.70	3400	$4857	6
B	.80	3200	4000	1
C	.90	4200	4667	4
D	1.00	4200	4200	3
E	1.10	5200	4727	5
F	1.20	5000	4167	2
G	1.30	5200	4000	1

appear very efficient and are ranked as high-potential participants in the preferred provider organization.

The use of the Medicare Case-Mix Index, as mentioned previously, must be done with care and its users must recognize all of the inherent limitations associated with it. Also, the CMI does not consider quality of care. Judgments about the qualitative nature of medical services provided must be made.

Assessment of hospital efficiency and the selection of institutions to participate in preferred provider organizations is clearly an inexact art. The tools and approaches discussed here have been reviewed only in a summary fashion to highlight some of the approaches being utilized as well as those that might be considered in the future. Some of the mechanisms presently being used to select physicians have been or could be used for the identification of preferred hospitals.

The Greater Baltimore Preferred Provider Organization uses hospital-specific information acquired by the Maryland Health Services Cost Review Commission (Table 5-7). Emerging PPOs may also use Delmarva's NAP methodology to identify facilities that report low levels of non acute days. As for the process suggested earlier for physicians, it would seem particularly meaningful to require applicant institutions to allow non acute profiles to be conducted by a PPO as part of the application process.

As competition between PPOs and other alternative delivery systems increases, it can be anticipated that the mechanisms outlined in this chapter will be accorded greater scrutiny and possible use.

PAYMENT ARRANGEMENTS

Earlier discussions have illustrated that certain provider payment approaches place constructive incentives on physicians and hospitals to control the cost of

Table 5-7 Hospital Efficiency Indicators as Measured by Days Above Average (DAA)

Days Above Average Report

Maryland
Health Services Cost Review Commission
Data Period = 1980 Data
Pay Source = All
Hospital: XXXX

	Hospital's		Region's		Days Above
DRG	PAT.	LOS	PAT.	LOS	Average
307	96	10.59	1086	7.56	291.2
380	62	9.77	1219	5.69	253.0
305	309	4.39	6797	3.74	201.4

Days Above Average
(Efficiency in Delivery of Care) Equals
Hospital's Length of Stay Minus
Region's Times Hospital's Patients;
Unusual Patient Cases Eliminated from Calculations

Source: Alvin D. Ankrum, *Analyzing Hospital Utilization and Efficiency* (Baltimore, Md.: Baltimore City Professional Standards Review Organization, February 1981).

medical care. The purpose of this section is not to provide a comprehensive treatise on all of these payment methods; rather, it is to explore creative ways that payment arrangements can be used to form the foundation of practical incentive programs for physicians and, to a lesser extent, hospitals. Before these incentives are considered, however, it is appropriate to review the use of discounts with respect to physician fees and hospital payment arrangements, and the extent to which these can be considered mechanisms for enhancing PPO cost efficiency.

Discounts and Physician Payment Mechanisms

Knowledgeable PPO participants recognize that discounted physician fees may not, in reality, be discounts at all. If a payment system is structured around the UCR reimbursement approach, physician payment is usually limited to a certain percentile of the usual, customary, and reasonable reimbursement provided physicians in a given geographical area for the procedures or services under consideration. Preferred provider organizations incorporating a maximum physician payment schedule linked to the 90th percentile of UCR may, at first, appear to be offering a 10 percent discount. In reality, however, the use of the 90th percentile may serve to increase fees. Increases will occur in an environment where the large majority of physicians routinely charge less than the 90th percentile. The most bizarre scenario would be a situation in which, prior to PPO involvement, all of the physicians associated with a preferred provider organization reported fees equal to the 50th percentile. The use of the 90th percentile, in this example, would actually offer an incentive for increasing the fees of those medical participants.

A similar analogy can be drawn for the use of the Relative Value Scale (RVS). The dollar multiplier attached to the RVS may be 20 percent less than the multiplier used by the physician community. The tendency, again, is to assume that this multiplier produces a 20 percent discount. However, for physicians already charging fees 30 percent below the community average, the utilization of such a multiplier offers an inflationary posture.

Preferred provider organizations have the opportunity to avoid the natural questions surrounding physician fee discounts by incorporating two features used by the Physicians' Alliance for Medical Excellence (Lexington, Kentucky). These two features have enhanced the marketing capabilities of the preferred provider organization. The Physicians' Alliance froze all physician fees until the end of its first fiscal year, October 31, 1983. The second unique feature of this preferred provider organization is that future fee increases for the 1984 fiscal year were limited to an increase that does not exceed the regional consumer price index.

Cost-Containment Features of Hospital Payment Methods

PPOs use three basic arrangements for paying hospitals: billed charges, per diems, and payments per admission.

The most common arrangement is billed charges (with a discount) followed by the all-inclusive payment for each day of care. Payment per case or admission is rare, although some purchasers have negotiated all-inclusive payment levels for high-cost services (such as coronary bypass procedures). Others, like Blue Cross/Blue Shield of Virginia, use payment per confinement as the PPO hospital payment method.

Billed Charges

Payment based on billed charges offers little, if any, incentive for serious cost control. Extended lengths of stay and excessive ancillary service usage are two costly physician behaviors tolerated by this payment method. From the perspective of a participating facility, this is the least risky and, indeed, preferred method of reimbursement; to a purchaser, though, the method merely perpetuates many of the financing problems that have produced the medical inflation problem of the 1980s.

Per Diem Payment

Unlike billed charges, all-inclusive payment for each day of care offers incentives for efficient daily hospital performance. This payment method shifts some of the financial risk from the purchaser to the provider of care, in this case the hospital, and in so doing stimulates greater cost consciousness. Yet it is important to note that the hospital has only a limited incentive and ability to act on that incentive. First, per diem payment does not financially penalize an institution for excessive lengths of stay; they are merely reimbursed. In an economic sense, a hospital receives no financial compensation for diligently policing its medical staff. On the contrary, it may frequently suffer the consequences of doing so. Organizational behavior in such an environment is predictable.

A hospital does receive a reward if it can control the costs of care rendered during each day of a patient's stay. Managerial efficiency plays a part, but the largest element of cost is beyond the scope of most hospitals' control: costly ancillary services ordered by physicians.

Per diem reimbursement, then, does provide theoretical incentives for cost-efficient behavior. Yet the individual hospital may have virtually no immediate control over this cost. Facilities able to reap the reward of per diem reimbursement are those having (1) a highly efficient medical staff, (2) a committed medical staff that aggressively works with or expels physicians who are inefficient, cost-escalating practitioners, or (3) the good fortune of a generous per diem that allows physician inefficiency to occur without financial distress being placed on the hospital.

One of the risks a hospital also faces with per diem reimbursement is case-mix imbalance. The daily cost of caring for a patient in intensive care is substantially greater than the cost of a routine pediatric surgical case. It is common for this risk to be at least partially avoided by the negotiation of individual per diems for major service areas: intensive care, burn care, medical cases, surgical cases, etc.

From a purchaser's point of view, per diem reimbursement is attractive because it essentially caps the daily cost of ancillary services. The obvious danger in its use concerns lengths of stay. Per diem payment without concurrent utilization review or assurances of length of stay control is an invitation to cost escalation.

AWARE, the PPO program offered by Blue Cross and Blue Shield of Minnesota (BCBSM), has employed a unique per diem payment approach designed to address the hospital and purchaser concerns discussed previously and, further, to do so while providing economic incentives to participating hospitals.[8] This payment arrangement is formulated on negotiated payment per day and negotiated length of stay for individual health service categories:

1. Obstetrical
2. Medical
3. Surgical
4. Nervous/Mental

5. Chemical Dependency
6. Heart Surgery
7. Diagnostic Heart Procedures
8. Hemodialysis
9. Spinal Fusion
10. Kidney Transplant
11. Bone Marrow Transplant
12. Uretero-Ileostomy
13. Hyperbaric Oxygenation
14. Radical Pancreatico-Duodenectomy
15. Pelvic Evisceration
16. Malignant Neoplasms of Blood and Lymphatic Systems

The 16 per diem payments and lengths of stay are negotiated between BCBSM and individual acute care facilities and included in the contractual agreement between the two. Such prospectively defined expectations are, in and of themselves, unique.

A contractual provision specifies that hospitals will be financially affected, positively or negatively, by length of stay changes. This legal provision states that at the end of a participation period, BCBSM will calculate an inpatient length of stay settlement for each of the 16 health service categories. This settlement will be equal to the difference between the actual length of stay and the negotiated length of stay (by each category) multiplied by the negotiated payment per day; it is multiplied again by the total number of inpatient admissions in each health service category:

$$ILOSS = (ALOS - NLOS \times NPPD \times ADM)$$

where:

ILOSS	=	Inpatient length of stay settlement, in dollars
ALOS	=	Actual length of stay
NLOS	=	Negotiated length of stay
NPPD	=	Negotiated payment per day
ADM	=	Number of admissions for the particular health service category

The hospital receives a cash incentive for those health service categories in which the actual length of stay is less than the negotiated length of stay. This cash payment is equal to 50 percent of the ILOSS value. If the actual length of stay for a health service category is above the NLOS, the hospital is contractually obligated to pay Blue Cross/Blue Shield of Minnesota 50 percent of the ILOSS.

An example can help illustrate how this incentive would operate. Table 5-8 contains assumptions for two common hospital health service categories: Medicine and Obstetrics. The actual length of stay for medical patients has been .5 days below the negotiated length of stay, resulting in a cash incentive payment of $13,750 for the hospital. The reverse is true for obstetrics; the actual average stay was .5 day above that negotiated, producing a cash payment from the hospital of $11,250.

Payment Per Admission

Hospital reimbursement per admission can assume two general forms. It can be adjusted for major diagnostic groups (DRG-type payment) or it may be an unadjusted average payment for each case, regardless of the diagnostic condition of the patient and/or the services provided to the patient. Payment per admission serves as an incentive toward efficient hospital behavior because it extends financial rewards to those facilities that deal seriously with the difficult task of controlling length of stay. This form of hospital payment also encourages hospitals and their medical staffs to address the fundamental underlying issue of "hospital" inefficiency, i.e., physician practice patterns. Hospitals, literally, cannot afford physicians with inefficient styles of practice. Such physicians, under this form of payment, can produce financial difficulties for the hospital in the short run. In the longer term, they disrupt the ability of a hospital to

---

Table 5-8 Assumptions and Calculations of Hospital Financial Incentive, Blue Cross and Blue Shield of Minnesota PPO (AWARE)

Service	Assumptions	
	Medicine	Obstetrics
NLOS	5.8	3.5
ALOS	5.3	4.0
NPPD	550	450
ADM	100	100

Calculations

Medicine ILOSS	$= (5.3 - 5.8) \times \$550 \times 100$
	$= \$27,500$
	Hospital Incentive $= .50 \times \$27,500$
	$= \$13,750$
Obstetrics ILOSS	$= (4.0 - 3.5) \times \$450 \times 100$
	$= \$22,500$
	Hospital Incentive $= .50 \times \$22,500$
	$= -\$11,250$

maintain its association with alternative delivery systems (PPOs, HMOs) in which cost efficiency is a high priority.

Payment per admission allows purchasers to share the financial risk of care with PPO providers. Further, institutional providers are confronted with financial incentives to undertake sweeping changes that are designed to produce greater physician efficiency.

The financial risk associated with this form of payment is significant enough to discourage involvement by hospitals with little or no ability to meet the challenges it presents. Those able to meet these challenges, however, may find the reimbursement method particularly appealing.

One would expect purchasers to welcome, with open arms, payment per admission. It shifts risk; it instills certain incentives; it aids budgeting. Adoption of this payment approach should gain momentum as the PPO movement matures. But adoption is likely to occur only when purchasers are assured that (1) negotiated payment levels are lean, not inflated, and (2) that adequate controls exist to keep patients out of the hospital in the first place.

The preceding cursory discussion of hospital payment methods in PPOs should leave the reader with at least one major impression: hospitals have relatively little control, in the short run, over how efficiently they perform. Stated simply, they lack sufficient enough control to dramatically alter physician practice styles in a short period of time. This implies that per diem and per admission payment methods will not meet their full efficiency potential until these payment approaches can be augmented so that physicians are financially affected by the efficiency or inefficiency of their practice styles.

The RFP: A Strategy for Negotiating Hospital Payment Levels

Regardless of the payment approach used by a PPO, certain tactical tools can be used to ensure that the most cost-efficient level of payment or discount is obtained.

One tool used by select preferred arrangements has been the Request For Proposal (RFP). The primary purpose of an RFP is to present hospitals with the requirements for PPO participation and afford them the opportunity to stipulate the level of discount and/or fee level they may find comfortable. In the proper environment, the RFP can serve equally the interests of both the hospital and the preferred provider organization. The hospital, with a knowledge of its own level of efficiency and inefficiency, can propose a payment structure that is both competitive and consistent with the financial needs of the institution.

Common sense suggests that a PPO will receive the greatest advantages from the RFP method in those health care systems characterized by strong competitive elements. Low hospital occupancies, strong interhospital competition, and the articulation of serious interest in PPO participation by major purchasers seem to place constructive pressure on hospitals to present highly competitive bids within the context of the RFP process.

One community that has effectively used the Request For Proposal method is San Diego.[9] The San Diego Foundation for Medical Care, which developed the San Diego Preferred Provider Organization, notified hospitals in San Diego County that maximum hospital participation would be limited to 30 percent of all inpatient facilities in the service area. The existence of strong competitive forces resulted in highly competitive proposals allowing the San Diego Preferred Provider Organization to pass along, on average, a reported 30 percent discount to participating purchasers. In this particular instance, the RFP method helped to produce cost controls which may have exceeded those that would have been proposed directly by the PPO entity.

The components of the RFP issued by the San Diego Preferred Provider Organization provide a useful framework for other preferred arrangements. These included:

- The Preferred Provider Organization program was designed to involve any and all third party payors and the medical panel consisted of 1,600 physicians. Potential institutional providers were informed that contracts with hospitals would be limited to only 30 percent of all hospitals in the metropolitan area.

- The RFP stated that cost containment would be the central feature of the PPO's operation. Both physicians and hospitals would be required to participate in the private sector utilization review program known as the Coalition Action Program (CAP). The CAP program provides major San Diego area employers with utilization review services focused heavily on preadmission certification and concurrent review.

- Hospitals were also informed that compensation would be based on a flat per diem charge for each patient day of inpatient service. This per diem charge was to be determined by the hospital and included in its response to the proposal.

- Certain diagnoses and procedures were excluded from those that would be based on the per diem. These included burn care, diagnostic admissions for cardiac catheterization, neonatal intensive care services, open heart surgery, and normal deliveries. Hospitals wishing to provide the last three items on a preferred provider basis were asked to submit a separate per diem for neonatal intensive care services, a separate DRG-based payment bid for elective open heart surgery regardless of length of stay, and a separately identified bid for obstetrical services, again, regardless of length of stay.

- The procedures for responding to the Request For Proposals were also identified for prospective institutional participants.

The RFP was sent to all institutions in the immediate metropolitan area along with a specimen of the contract that would be executed upon acceptance of individual proposals.

It seems clear that the RFP method employed by the San Diego PPO measurably assisted cost control in that organization. The RFP was of such usefulness because of the highly competitive environment in the San Diego metropolitan area. During 1980, two-thirds of the facilities operated at occupancy rates below 70 percent. This situation, coupled with several other important competitive characteristics, made the RFP process useful. Communities where interhospital competition is nonexistent or very limited will find the RFP process to have far less potential.

INCENTIVES FOR EFFICIENT PHYSICIAN BEHAVIOR

A physician incentive program can be defined as an arrangement in which physicians are periodically given financial compensation for efficient practice behavior. The ongoing nature of such incentive programs suggests that the financial incentives would be provided on a monthly or other short-term, periodic basis. However, there do not appear to be any programs providing short-term incentives. Those that do provide financial incentives do so, or plan to do so, using incentive pools. A physician incentive pool can be described as a lump sum of money acquired over a lengthy period of time, perhaps a year, which is redistributed to providers on the basis of individual or collective efficiency as judged by predefined criteria. The San Diego Committee for Affordable Health Care, Independence Medical Systems in the Clearwater, Florida, area, and Virginia's KeyCare are programs with plans to develop incentive pool arrangements.

In the summer of 1983, the San Diego Committee for Affordable Health Care received a $100,000 grant from the Robert Wood Johnson Foundation to proceed with the planning and development of a community-based preferred provider organization. A central component of the application submitted to the Robert Wood Johnson Foundation was the proposed development of a financial incentive system.[10] The San Diego Committee for Affordable Health Care hopes to reduce medical costs by offering such incentives to physicians whose fees do not exceed defined target figures. Providers whose costs of providing care are less than or equal to those computed by a detailed formula will receive a portion of the savings generated by the preferred provider organization. This program is expected to be operational in 1985.

Independence Medical Systems (IMS) originally anticipated the initiation of a similar physician incentive pool. The principals behind the investor-owned IMS have strong health maintenance organization backgrounds. Their previous

HMO experience with incentive pools initially led them in the direction of a similar arrangement for PPO physicians. Incentives to physicians were to be provided on a deferred income basis. The objective of such an approach was to provide financial incentives that reshape physician behavior in a fashion consistent with cost efficiency while, at the same time, maximizing the tax advantages of the financial incentive. As of mid-1984, however, the developing PPO has temporarily deferred the incentive pool in favor of options to purchase PPO "stock" at a designated point in the future. Physicians found such an opportunity more appealing than the earlier incentive arrangement.

The PPO product begun by Blue Cross/Blue Shield of Virginia, KeyCare, has established the Professional Provider Incentive Program.[11] The principal goal of the program is to financially reward physicians for reducing hospital admissions and inpatient days. Participating physicians have agreed to accept a fee schedule that is less than UCR. To the extent that the program goals are met, providers will receive incentive payments up to the amount they would have received under the UCR schedule. The incentive payments will be calculated on the basis of services provided by each professional provider within a calendar year. The methodology used to calculate physician incentive payments more heavily weights services provided in an outpatient setting than those provided on an inpatient basis. The KeyCare program began in mid-1983. The first incentive payments are expected in April 1985.

There are two immediately identifiable problems with the incentive pool approach. The first is that incentives provided semiannually or annually may be so infrequent as to minimize their impact. The second may be even more difficult to address. A preferred provider organization must generate surplus funds to build the incentive pool. Many PPOs, like those established individually by hospitals or jointly by hospitals and physicians, do not have this capacity. Situations in which physicians are paid on a fee-for-service basis and hospitals are paid on a basis of billed charges simply do not provide the financial avenue for effectively establishing incentive pool arrangements.

It would appear that serious incentive pools can be established only in environments in which the PPO or its providers have assumed some degree of risk. If hospitals and/or hospital-based preferred provider organizations are paid on a per admission or per diem basis, high levels of efficiency may allow surplus revenue to accrue, providing the foundation for the incentive pool.

There is a growing trend for purchasers to encourage greater risk sharing and, accordingly, the use of per diem and per admission reimbursement arrangements. In the following sections, two ways are suggested that these types of payment might potentially be used to serve as incentives for efficient physician behavior. The first proposed approach is called The Physician Incentive Reporting Program; the second is termed the Physician Incentive Account.

The Physician Incentive Reporting Program (PIRP)

The Physician Incentive Reporting Program recognizes that hospitals paid on a per diem or per admission basis incur a direct financial risk. Efficient physicians minimize this risk and may even produce a net surplus; inefficient physicians maximize the risk and likely produce net losses. Given such a situation, it would appear advantageous for hospitals to reward financially those practitioners who practice their art efficiently. One approach is The Physician Incentive Reporting Program (PIRP) (see Figure 5-1) in which a hospital offers individual physicians an annual incentive payment that parallels their practice efficiency. The annual incentive has a more timely impact than an annual incentive pool because individual physicians are informed weekly of their practice behavior and level of incentive. The components of the PIRP are as follows:

1. A preferred provider organization pays for hospital services through the use of prospectively negotiated per diem or per admission payments.
2. The hospital, in turn, agrees to divide with physicians the surplus generated by efficient practice behavior.
3. Surpluses or losses are determined by comparing actual billed charges for each individual patient with revenue received for that patient from the preferred provider organization (per diem/per admission).
4. Profits are not directly given to the physician. Rather, a computerized report is established to record the surplus/loss resulting from the practice patterns and efficiency of individual physicians.
5. Individual physicians are provided a weekly report of underpayments and overpayments. This information indicates the cumulative amount due the physician at the end of the payment cycle.
6. The hospital pays the physician on an annual basis.

The PIRP acknowledges that even efficient physicians will generate billed charges that periodically exceed PPO payments for certain diagnostic groups or patients of a certain severity of illness. The cumulative reporting of underpayments and overpayments to the facility provides the mechanism for paying a periodic financial incentive representing the net level of efficiency demonstrated by individual practitioners. Table 5-9 illustrates the kind of information that would be collected and reported weekly to a physician. This table also hints at the influence such information might have on overall physician behavior.

This system could work with either per diem or per admission payment to the hospital from the preferred provider organization. Per diem payment would produce the least amount of risk since the level of total payment would fluctuate with the length of stay. Per case payment, on the other hand, would be irrespective of length of stay and transfer a greater level of risk to participating facilities.

Figure 5-1 The Physician Incentive Reporting Program

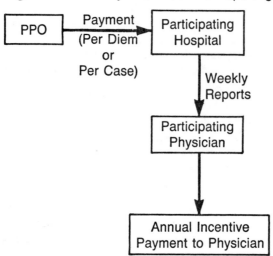

A major problem with the PIRP centers around those physicians who persistently produce underpayments for the hospital. The natural question facing an administrator can be phrased as follows: "I can give incentives to efficient providers, but can I take away money from inefficient ones?" The probable answer is "no." One solution, however, would be to carry over a certain level of inefficiency from one year to the next. An example illustrates this particular point. Assume that John Q. Doctor, discussed in Table 5-9, had concluded the year 1982 with a total underpayment of $5,000. The underpayment of $5,000 indicates that his practice style was less efficient than expected. Assume also that the hospital in which he practices has no ability to charge the physician for his behavior. Indeed, rarely would an institution undertake such politically volatile action. The hospital, though, may have policies that allow for the carryover of a certain level of underpayment. If this carryover level were set, for example, at 50 percent, John Q. Doctor would have begun 1983 with an existing underpayment level of $2,500.

The Physician Incentive Account (PIA)

Another approach to providing incentives for efficient physician behavior is the Physician Incentive Account (PIA) (see Figure 5-2). The Physician Incentive Account is directly established and maintained by the preferred provider organization. For each hospitalized patient, the PPO credits the attending physician's account with a prospectively determined amount. It is important to note that the

Table 5-9 The Physician Incentive Reporting Program: An Example

Physician: John Q. Doctor, M.D.
Hospital: Doctor's Medical Center
Period: Nov. 19–Nov. 26, 1983

Patient Number	Length of Stay	Total Billed Charges	Expected/ Received Total pmt. to Hospital from PPO	Underpayment	Overpayment
A2103	4	$2700	2900	—	200
A2801	7	4200	4900	—	700
A2998	3	1700	1700	—	—
B0062	12	6400	4700	1700	—
C1111	5	2900	3400	—	500
C1250	9	5700	6500	—	600
C1397	9	7200	8500	—	1300
D1211	4	3900	2500	1400	—
D4222	5	3900	4400	—	500
TOTAL				3100	3800

For the above one week reporting period overpayment to the hospital because of your practice patterns totaled $800.

Cumulative overpayment to the hospital for the year to day (Jan. 1983 to Nov. 26, 1983) totals $11,002. If this trend continues, cumulative overpayment will total $12,002.38 by Dec. 31, 1983. Based on the Physician-Hospital Agreement covering the Physician Incentive Reporting Program, your annual incentive payment will be $6,001.19.

physician, not the hospital, is the initial recipient of PPO payment for hospital care. This amount may or may not be DRG specific. It may be per diem based or it may be per admission. At the conclusion of the patient's (successful) hospital episode, the hospital bills the physician's account for the total (or discounted total) of billed charges generated by that physician. The PPO, as the administrator of the account, remits the prescribed amount. The preferred provider organization serves as a financial intermediary for the transaction, transferring funds from the Physician Incentive Account directly to the hospital. The PIA would be most appropriately initiated by physician-sponsored PPOs. One West Michigan PPO in the process of development has tentative plans to employ the PIA, using DRG-based payments, for the 50 most frequent diagnoses/procedures.[12]

The Physician Incentive Account affords several advantages for participating physicians and the preferred provider organization. The first advantage concerns the influence that such an incentive account might have on the behavior of physicians. The financial risk assumed by physicians in this type of payment

Figure 5-2 The Physician Incentive Account

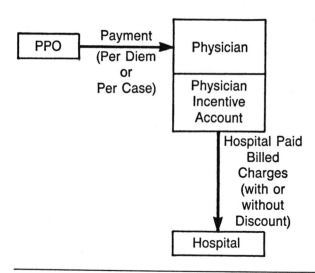

arrangement suggests that increased practice efficiency would result as a matter of necessity. The PIA also provides significant cash flow improvement possibilities. The costliness of hospital care makes it realistically possible for individual accounts to quickly approach several thousands or even hundreds of thousands of dollars. Physician cash flow can be maximized by ensuring payment from the PPO to the physician in a very timely manner while, simultaneously, delaying payments from the PIA to the hospital.

The enhancement of physician cash flow raises the question of the relationship between individual hospitals and the preferred provider organization. Under the scenario presented here, it is quite possible that a preferred provider organization would not execute contracts with hospitals. Contracts would be entered into only with physicians using the Physician Incentive Account approach for payment. Physicians would be free to use any facility they wished, reaping either the financial rewards or penalties of their behavior. The financial incentives of the PIA approach could be expected to link physician inpatient practice patterns to lower-cost, high-quality facilities.

One of the difficult issues to resolve with respect to the Physician Incentive Account is the way in which the payment to the physician would be determined. One method that might be appropriate is as follows:

1. The preferred provider organization would establish a defined length of stay for individual DRGs. The defined length of stay might be consistent with the 50th percentile of all lengths of stay for the individual DRG as

reported by certain abstract services, e.g., the Commission on Professional and Hospital Activities (PAS Program).

2. The per diem to be credited to the PIA could be structured in either of two ways: it could equal the average for all hospitals in the community or it could equal the average hospital daily charge at the particular hospital being used by a particular physician. The first approach would encourage physicians to use cost-efficient inpatient facilities; the second recognizes the political problems inherent in such an effort.

3. The preferred provider organization would determine whether any discount would be appropriate.

4. Payment to an individual physician, i.e., payment to that physician's PIA, would be the product of the average hospital per diem multiplied by the average length of stay at the 50th percentile as reported (by PAS) for the individual diagnosis-related group.

The concept of the Physician Incentive Account is not one to be considered casually by physicians. Any physician pursuing involvement in a PIA arrangement with a preferred provider organization should do so only after reviewing past hospital practice patterns. The physician is at financial risk in this approach.

INFORMATION FEEDBACK SYSTEMS: PSYCHIC INCENTIVE SYSTEMS

The Physician Incentive Account is one conceptual approach to altering inpatient physician practice behavior through the use of economic incentives and disincentives. It can be argued, however, that the mere provision of meaningful information can help shape efficient practice patterns. The provision of timely information on the efficiency of a physician, as compared with other physicians, can facilitate cost-efficient practice behavior by providing a psychic incentive.

Three preferred provider organizations have developed information feedback systems of interest. One, a West Coast preferred provider arrangement jointly established by a multihospital system and its physicians, provides participating physicians with a daily statement on the medical chart of each patient. This chart identifies the diagnosis (DRG) of the patient, the expected average length of stay for that particular DRG, and the average cost for that condition. This information is compared with the current number of days the patient has been in the hospital and the accumulated charges. Table 5-10 presents information that might be provided to PPO physicians in an information feedback system.

Comprehensive Medical Care Affiliates, Inc. (CompMed) is a nonprofit preferred provider organization wholly owned by the St. John Medical Center in Kansas City, Missouri. This organization has established an information feedback

Table 5-10 Information Feedback System for Physicians, West Coast
PPO

DRG:249; Diabetes, Age 36 or Older

Expected Average Length of Stay: 10 days	Current Number of Days Used: 4 days
Average Charges per Day: $400	Current Charges per Day (average): $300
Average Cost per Stay: $4,000	Cumulative Charges: $1,200

system that provides physicians with a daily statement of the cumulative charge
to each patient. This system does not approach the detail employed by the West
Coast preferred provider organization. CompMed officials believe, though, that
this system has influenced physician behavior. During the first two months of
operation PPO patients were experiencing an average length of stay .7 of one
day less than comparable patients. In October 1983, overall savings generated
by PPO physicians were estimated to be 8 percent less than the cost of care
rendered to non-PPO patients.

Physician-specific Non Acute Profiles, discussed previously, are serving as
the basis of a feedback system for medical practitioners affiliated with KeyCare,
the PPO developed by Blue Cross and Blue Shield of Virginia.[13] The system
periodically provides physicians with a comparative analysis of both the extent
and reason for nonacute utilization.

The Delmarva Foundation for Medical Care has studied the impact such feedback can have on physician practice behavior. The Foundation has produced
three important findings. First, it has observed that physicians agree with the
objectively applied criteria used to determine if a day of care is nonacute. Also,
because of this agreement, physicians involved in Delmarva's review program
concur with the findings resulting from the use of the criteria. Most important,
physician hospitalization practice behavior undergoes rapid and noticeable change
when statistical NAP comparisons are presented to physicians. The Foundation
has persistently observed immediate length of stay reductions of ½ and 1 day
at those facilities involved in Delmarva's programs. Over a two-year period,
one facility in the Delmarva service area recorded a reduction from 7 days to
5½ days in the average length of stay.

These findings suggest that this particular type of feedback has unparalleled
potential for facilitating the cost-control performance of PPOs, like KeyCare,
which employ it.

UTILIZATION REVIEW

The predominant approach to cost containment in preferred provider organizations has been the implementation of aggressive utilization review programs.

The popularity of utilization control mechanisms has resulted from the inability of preferred provider organizations to exercise meaningful control over the selection of physicians or to implement tangible, productive incentive systems. Utilization review programs will be one of the predominant factors in determining the survival of preferred provider organizations. In the absence of prospective selection systems or strong incentive arrangements, utilization review represents the single most important component for both success and survival.

Preferred provider organizations have implemented a wide variety of utilization review controls. There are those PPOs that mandate strong controls for all participating groups. Others allow individual purchasers to select and choose those utilization controls considered most appropriate.

Utilization review programs are not new. They have been around for decades. The demands articulated by the purchaser sector, and response to these demands by preferred provider organizations, however, have injected new life into a process that can only be characterized in retrospect as having been mediocre in nature and of very questionable effectiveness. The recognition that PPO survival depends heavily on the success of utilization review programs has measurably contributed to the renewed interest and emerging effectiveness of utilization control.[14]

Figure 5-3 The Conceptual Relationship Between Volume of Services and Patient Outcome

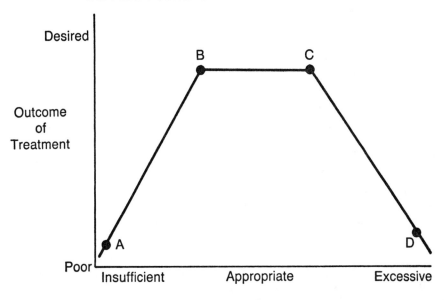

Volume of Service Delivered

The objective of the review process is primarily education. Physician performance is compared with expected standards. Those physicians persistently at variance with quality and efficiency standards are identified and, through numerous mechanisms, encouraged to, simply, "clean up their act." Figure 5-3 illustrates the conceptual nature of the review process. It attempts to bring physicians whose performance is characterized as poor (point A) or by excessive use of resources (points C and D) to a level of desired medical outcome using appropriate amounts of services (point B).

Utilization control programs are being implemented in various combinations by preferred arrangements. PPO programs include preadmission certification, admission review, mandatory second opinion, concurrent length of stay analysis, retrospective review, and ambulatory services review. The following sections will highlight the principal components of these very important control mechanisms.

Preadmission Certification

Preadmission certification is a screening process that filters out those patients for which inpatient services are not required. The intention of this review mechanism is to ensure that those persons hospitalized require the intensive and costly services provided within the walls of acute care institutions. Typically, the preadmission certification process is applied to all elective hospital admissions or to more focused groups of admission/diagnostic categories frequently associated with inappropriate hospitalization.

The Southern California-based, physician-owned California Preferred Professionals (CPP) has developed a set of utilization guidelines that includes a list of over 1,000 medical procedures that must be performed on an outpatient basis.[15] There are also over 25 procedures that require preadmission certification before hospital admission. Blue Cross of California's PPO, Prudent Buyer Plan, defines three categories of diagnoses and procedures considered to require preadmission review.[16] Category I includes procedures that require prior authorization to determine the medical necessity of inpatient care. Category II includes procedures and diagnoses generally performed on an outpatient basis. Any of these procedures performed on an inpatient basis require that documentation of extra risk factors be presented to guarantee payment if hospital admission occurs. The third category of diagnoses and procedures are those typically excluded from Blue Cross benefit agreements (cosmetic surgery).

Preadmission certification is a step-by-step process involving an individual patient's physician and the reviewing entity. Commonly, the attending physician, or the physician's representative, contacts the reviewing body, informing them of the admission and the reasons for the admission. The reviewing body, such as a foundation for medical care, considers the request for admission, comparing it with physician-developed criteria utilized by the review organization. The admission is subsequently considered to be medically necessary and appropriate or to be inappropriate. The preadmission certification process is usually performed on a timely basis with decisions being rendered frequently within 24 hours.

There are times when an admission is not certified. In these instances, the physician is encouraged to utilize outpatient services as the mechanism for providing medical care to the patient. In instances of disagreement between the physician and the reviewing body, an appeals procedure and/or grievance mechanism becomes operational. These vary from review body to review body. The appeal process always involves a physician's peers. In instances when a request for admission is ultimately denied, the patient is issued a letter advising him or her of the determination. Depending on the arrangement, the patient may be partially or wholly responsible for the cost of hospital care delivered when certification for admission is withheld.

Preadmission certification has been demonstrated to be an extremely effective and cost-efficient tool for restraining medical expenditures. In 1982, the San Diego Employers Health Cost Coalition initiated private sector review for coalition members. After one year, the program, which included both preadmission and current utilization review, produced a significant reduction in the use of inpatient hospital services. Pacific Southwest Airlines reported that the number of patient days per 1,000 employees/dependents was reduced by 10 percent within one year after the initiation of the program.[17] The Medical Care Foundation of Sacramento, California, instituted the Certified Hospital Admission Program in 1972 in order to reduce inpatient hospital admissions. In the first year of operation the CHAP program saved an estimated $3.50 for each dollar spent to conduct the review.[18]

Second Opinion Programs

Second opinion programs represent a type of preadmission review. Second opinion programs recognize that unusually high levels of unnecessary surgery may occur for selected conditions or diagnoses. Like the general preadmission certification review program, second opinion efforts can be either generalized or focused; that is, second opinions may be required for all elective surgeries (generalized) or for only a select set of conditions found to be frequently abused (focused). Second opinion programs can be costly and expensive particularly in a generalized program in which one or more second opinion may be rendered.

Second opinion programs operated by utilization review bodies or sponsored by major purchasers have produced the observation that effectiveness is closely related to (1) the mandatory nature of the program and (2) the focusing of the program only on those conditions most likely to be abused. A study published by the Health Care Financing Administration in 1981 concluded that "the estimates of program benefit and costs yields a benefit cost ratio of 2.63. That is, for every one dollar of cost incurred, two dollars and sixty-three cents in benefits occurred. The demonstrated cost savings potential of a mandatory second opinion program justifies the inclusion of such programs in the array of cost-containment initiatives already adopted or under consideration as a means of controlling the rise in medical care cost."[19]

Admission Review

Preadmission certification, even under the most ideal circumstances, is not always able to screen each and every patient admission. For a variety of reasons, patients may be admitted for elective or other services without the admission screening. Admission review is a concurrent procedure that complements the preadmission certification process. It is a process usually conducted within 24 hours of an admission, rendering a decision about the appropriateness of an admission. If a patient is found to have been inappropriately admitted, the patient, after consultation with the physician, is discharged to a more appropriate level of service or, when disagreement occurs with the physician, the appeals process is initiated. For those admissions found to be appropriate and necessary, the concurrent length of stay procedure described below becomes operational.

Concurrent Length of Stay Review

Concurrent length of stay review is an evaluation and monitoring process which attempts to ensure that a patient's length of stay is the shortest possible but most appropriate for the conditions surrounding the patient's admission.

A typical concurrent length of stay process begins at the assignment of an expected length of stay. The assignment is performed by a nurse coordinator, using length of stay guidelines established by a physician review body. The length of stay criteria vary across review groups, though, commonly, the diagnosis/procedure lengths of stay generated by The Commission on Professional and Hospital Activities are used.

At periodic checkpoints during a patient's hospital stay, the nurse coordinator reviews the patient's progress and need for continued hospitalization. This is accomplished by comparing documentation in the patient's record to continued stay criteria of the review body. In some cases, a patient's condition will require a hospital stay that exceeds the expected length of stay established upon admission. When appropriate, additional days are approved. However, in instances where the review nurse cannot certify continued hospitalization, physician advisers are involved in the review process.

Unresolved disagreements between the attending physician and the review body are channeled through an appeals process. Patients are typically notified that they may be financially responsible for hospital stays that are not ultimately approved.

Like preadmission certification and other review processes, concurrent length of stay review is effective only when it is applied seriously. One of the critical aspects of this process concerns the establishment of diagnosis/procedure-specific length of stay. Very generous stay levels defeat the purpose of this review process. An example of an aggressive length of stay program will help put this process in an appropriate context. The Midwest Foundation for Medical Care (Cincinnati) uses the length of stay at the 50th percentile of the Professional Activities Study (PAS) as the norm for inpatient stays. The PAS information, which comes from Ann Arbor's Commission on Professional and Hospital Activities, is diagnosis, procedure, and age specific. The 50th percentile means that 50 percent of all patients admitted for a particular diagnosis have lengths of stay equal to or less than the particular length associated with the 50th percentile.

Physician practice patterns are monitored through the use of computer software developed by Stoner and Associates, a Cincinnati third party administrator. According to Stoner, the computer monitoring system compares the actual length of stay with that suggested by PAS for each admission. This difference—whether a positive or a negative number—is called the delta statistic. The delta statistic is determined by subtracting the PAS length of stay from the actual length of stay. The delta statistic is calculated for each admission.

The Delstat System calculates the mean and the standard deviation of the delta statistic for any group of admissions being studied. The mean delta statistic for any number or combination of admissions is a quantifiable value that can be identified, ranked, compared, and monitored over time.

The Delstat System using the delta statistic also provides a valid comparison between groups of admissions while accounting for differences in patient mix between these groups. Within the Delstat System, comparisons can be made between employer/carrier groups, medical specialties, and periods of time. Comparisons can also be made by determining the delta statistic for individual physicians and admissions by day of week.

The extensive nature of Midwest's data capabilities serves as a model for PPO concurrent review activities. Exhibit 5-2 outlines the data computerized for each concurrent review conducted by the organization. A vast number of highly specific comparisons and management reports may be generated by this system.

Retrospective Review: Inpatient and Outpatient

Retrospective review is an after-the-fact process designed to assess whether the care rendered to a patient was appropriate. This review is linked necessarily

Exhibit 5-2 Computerized Information Used by Midwest Foundation for
Medical Care in Concurrent Review Process

Patient Record Number	Final Diagnosis
Patient's Social Security Number	Secondary Diagnosis
Zip Code	PAS Days
Identifier-Surname	First Procedure Date
Nurse Coordinator	First Procedure Code
Sex	Discharge Status D/S
Age	Second Procedure Date
Admitting Date	Second Procedure Code
Hospital	Appeal
Type of Admission	Extension Days Attending
Admitting Physician	Extension Days Admitting
Physician Specialty	Extension Days MRC
Carrier/Employer	Days Saved
Consulting Physician	Discharge Date
Receipt Data	Total Authorized
Admitting Diagnosis	LOS
Specialty Code	

with the claims-processing function. From a cost-containment perspective, costly ancillary services and procedures are a major focus of this review activity. Even though an admission is justified and the patient's stay was within prescribed standards, the excessive and unnecessary use of costly ancillary services (and consultations) can measurably escalate the cost of a hospital stay. Further, the emphasis of PPOs on ambulatory services mandates that PPOs eventually incorporate ambulatory review mechanisms.

CONCLUSIONS

Until physician selection processes and incentive systems are refined, utilization review will remain the workhorse of cost control in preferred provider arrangements. There is a large body of information to support the contention that utilization review can be most effective. The experience of the San Diego Employers Health Cost Coalition, reported earlier in this chapter, is one example. Many others exist. The Iowa Foundation for Medical Care has been credited with a 9 percent decrease in patient days used per 1,000 Medicare beneficiaries and a 10 percent reduction in length of stay between 1976 and 1979. The same foundation's review program produced an 18.7 percent reduction in the number of hospital days used per 1,000 employees of Deere and Company resulting in a savings of over $10 for each $1 spent for review.[20]

The outcome of other utilization studies suggests that aggressive preadmission certification and concurrent review can establish savings that are 5 to 10 times the cost of incorporating utilization services. There can be no doubt that PPOs will increasingly adopt tight utilization control standards to produce savings for their clients and, in doing so, ensure the competitiveness of their programs.

NOTES

1. S. Brian Barger and David G. Hillman, "Cost Efficiency in Preferred Provider Organizations: Part II " *PPO Newsletter* 1, no. 3 (March 1984): 1+; S. Brian Barger and David G. Hillman, "Cost Efficiency in Preferred Arrangements: Part I " *PPO Newsletter* 1, no. 2 (February 1984): 1+.

2. Office of Health Maintenance Organizations, *Private Sector Investment in Health Maintenance Organizations: A Case Study of Venture Capital Financing* (Rockville, Md.: U.S. Department of Health and Human Services, July 1982).

3. P.J. Borchardt, "Non Acute Profiles: Evaluation of Physicians Non Acute Utilization of Hospital Resources," *Quality Review Bulletin* (November 1981): 21–26; P.J. Borchardt, "Effective Utilization Review: Non Acute Profiles and Intensive Review" (Paper delivered at the First National PPO Congress, Washington, D.C., January 10–11, 1984).

4. W.H. Kirby, *Proposal To Perform Intensified Review* (Baltimore: Health Management Services, Inc.) (Marketing information for clients).

5. Health Care Financing Administration, "Hospital Case Mix Indexes," *Federal Register* (September 1, 1983): 39647–39669.

6. J. Pettengill and J. Vertrees, "Reliability and Validity in Hospital Case Mix Measurement," *Health Care Financing Review* 4, no. 2 (December 1982): 101–128.

7. S. Brian Barger and David G. Hillman, *Preferred Provider Organizations and Grand Haven Michigan: A Feasibility Assessment* (Cincinnati, Oh.: Morgan Bigae Institute, June 1984), 19–22; Neil S. Fleming, "Rating Providers by Case-Mix Adjustment," *Business Insurance* (May 12, 1984): 43–44; P.D. Fox and J.J. Spies, "Alternative Delivery Systems: What Are the Risks?" *Business and Health* (January–February 1984): 8–9.

8. Blue Cross and Blue Shield of Minnesota, "Provider Service Agreement (Institutional)," in *National Conference on Preferred Product Development* (Chicago: Blue Cross and Blue Shield Association, September 1983).

9. San Diego Preferred Provider Organization, *Request for Proposal Concerning Hospital Services* (San Diego: San Diego PPO, March 30, 1983).

10. R.L. Rundle, "San Diego Employers Behind Push for Local PPO," *Business Insurance* (May 30, 1983): 16.

11. Blue Cross/Blue Shield of Virginia, "KeyCare Professional Provider Incentive Program," in *Proceedings of National Conference on Preferred Product Development* (Chicago: Blue Cross and Blue Shield Association, September 1983).

12. S. Brian Barger and David G. Hillman, *Preferred Provider Organizations and Grand Haven Michigan: A Feasibility Assessment* (Cincinnati, Oh.: Morgan Bigae Institute, June 1984), 88–90.

13. Blue Cross/Blue Shield of Virginia, "KeyCare Utilization Review Program," in *Proceedings of National Conference on Preferred Product Development* (Chicago: Blue Cross and Blue Shield Association, September 1983).

14. J.M. Perler, "Utilization Review for the PPO: The Ingredients of a Practical Plan for Concurrent Review," *Hospial Forum* 25 (November–December 1982): 23–25.

15. Suzanne Viau, *PPOs: State of the Art* (Washington, D.C.: Health Publishing Ventures, 1983), 25–26.

16. S.J. Tibbitts and A.J. Manzano, *Preferred Provider Organizations: An Executive Guide* (Chicago: Pluribus Press, 1984), 246–250.

17. Personal communication with Robert Colasanto, Director of Insurance and Employee Benefits, Pacific Southwest Airlines, June 1983.

18. Greater St. Louis Health Systems Agency, "Private Utilization Review Programs," in *Health Care Cost Management: A Review of Major Strategies* (St. Louis: St. Louis HSA, March 1982), 23.

19. M.L. Finkel, H.S. Richlin, and S.K. Parsons, *Eight Years Experience with a Second Opinion Elective Surgery Program: Utilization and Economic Analyses* (Baltimore: Health Care Financing Administration, March 1981), XV.

20. Iowa Foundation for Medical Care, *Marketing Briefs* (Des Moines, Ia.: 1981).

Part III

PPO Development: Technical and Organizational Approaches

Chapter 6

Assessing the Feasibility of Establishing a Preferred Provider Organization

Unlike health maintenance organizations, preferred provider development to date has not been heavily dependent upon extensive feasibility studies. The reasons for this are threefold. First, PPOs do not assume financial risks like those embodied in prepaid, capitated delivery systems. The relative lack of risk has allowed a more casual approach to PPO construction. Second, the health care marketplace has been generally receptive, at least in concept, to the emergence of preferred panel arrangements. And last, the technical tasks required for PPO development have been more easily integrated into the traditional practice of medicine and are of a less complex nature than HMO development.

This is not meant to suggest that feasibility studies have been unnecessary. On the contrary, preferred provider organizations in Kansas City and Birmingham, to name just a few, have conducted financial-oriented as well as more comprehensive feasibility assessments. Baptist Medical Center in Birmingham, Alabama, for example, used outside consultants to undertake a broad-based feasibility study to define the impact of a preferred provider organization on the hospital, focusing particularly on financial influence. This same feasibility study was also helpful in determining physician fee levels as well as the volume of PPO-related business that would be required to allow Baptist Medical Center to offer discounts.

PPO feasibility studies have also served other purposes. Perhaps one of the most important purposes of a feasibility study conducted by external consultants is to convince key hospital decision makers, such as hospital Boards of Trustees and senior medical staff members, that PPO development may be in the best interest of participating hospitals.

While feasibility assessment has been both relatively unnecessary and infrequent, there are clues strongly suggesting that, in the future, institutions participating in preferred provider organizations will need to seriously assess the feasibility of either developing and/or participating in a preferred provider or-

113

ganization. Why will the nonchalance of past feasibility assessment be inadequate in the future? There are several reasons. It is probable that preferred provider organizations will increasingly involve multiple medical facilities. This is in contrast to many of the recently developed preferred provider organizations that have utilized only one acute care facility. Greater geographic distribution and increased consumer choice results from multiple-hospital programs and significantly enhances the competitiveness of such PPOs.

The most obvious implication of multiple institutional involvement, however, is that the solicited patient pool may be divided among more institutions; the financial benefits to individual institutional participants will be fewer. Second, future PPO activity is likely to occur in less highly competitive geographic areas of the United States. This suggests that future PPO development activity will be greeted with less interest on the part of physicians and, possibly, hospitals. Additional resources will have to be devoted to the development of the preferred arrangement, thus increasing developmental costs as well as the time required to fully establish a PPO.

Third, demands from the purchaser sector will require preferred provider organizations to consider payment and reimbursement approaches that create a higher degree of financial risk. While many existing preferred provider organizations pay hospitals on the basis of billed charges, there is a growing momentum for payment based on per diems or payment per admission. Several Blue Cross/ Blue Shield plans have begun paying institutions in such ways: Blue Cross/Blue Shield plans of Minnesota, California, Virginia, and Kansas are each using payment systems that place individual hospitals at financial risk for the efficiency of care delivered. A fourth reason that PPO feasibility assessments will be necessary comes again from demand by the purchaser sector. Major purchasers have an interest in acquiring data that will demonstrate to them the utilization and cost-containment effectiveness of those PPOs in which they participate. Hospital-sponsored preferred provider organizations, as well as other types of PPOs, will, then, need sophisticated, costly data systems that are able to provide purchasers with diagnosis-specific information.

For these reasons future PPO activity will be more expensive to initiate and, because of different payment arrangements, will contain greater financial risks to participating hospitals and physicians. In such an environment, the ability to assess the probability of PPO effectiveness becomes essential.

PPO FEASIBILITY STUDIES: AN OVERVIEW

The feasibility of any particular endeavor is related to the desired outcome of that activity. In a similar way, the definition of PPO feasibility is individualized and directly associated with the goals and objectives that have been stated for that organization. The objective of one PPO might be merely to expand the market share and increase the competitiveness of participating institutions and medical practitioners. Other preferred provider organizations may be less concerned about competitiveness and more concerned about the impact the PPO has on the revenue and profit margin of its underwriters/investors/owners. There are clearly other types of objectives that preferred provider organizations may articulate.

Objectives

In general, PPO feasibility studies are mainly objective analyses containing some subjective components, and are designed to answer four key questions:

1. If a preferred provider organization is developed, will it achieve the objectives that have been stated for it?
2. Are there existing barriers to the development of this preferred provider organization?
3. Can these barriers be removed or at least minimized to allow the preferred provider organization to achieve a viable state of operation?
4. How will the resolution or elimination of such barriers affect the structure and direction that the preferred provider organization assumes?

The PPO Development Process

It is important, also, to note that the feasibility study is merely one part of a much longer process involved in PPO development. Once a particular preferred provider approach has been deemed feasible, the developing entity needs to undertake three additional processes: planning, development, and operation.

Planning, as the second of four major phases of PPO development, is characterized by refinement of some of the initial feasibility estimates, in particular those concerning financial matters.

The development phase involves the establishment of the legal PPO entity and is focused heavily on the development and consummation of contracts with physicians, hospitals, subscribing/purchaser groups and other subcontractors. Subcontractors would include groups performing some PPO function, e.g., those that might conduct utilization review or claims administration. It is during the development phase that a data system for utilization review, program monitoring, and management decision making is constructed. Marketing also begins in the development phase and is oriented toward key groups of purchasers or purchasing agents such as large self-funded employers, third party administrators, employee benefits brokers, and major insurance companies.

The concluding phase of PPO development is initial operation. This commences with the direct provision of medical services, as marketing continues. The PPO conducts all normal management, administration, and monitoring functions during this phase.

Exhibit 6-1 highlights the four principal phases of PPO development and the major characteristics of each phase.

Study Components

As noted in Exhibit 6-1, there are four components of a PPO feasibility study: legal, provider relations, marketing, and financial. Legal issues, including state laws, liability concerns, and general corporate law, form the foundation for the feasibility assessment. If such laws prohibit or create significant barriers to PPO development, further feasibility activities are of limited value. The willingness of physicians and hospitals to participate in the preferred arrangement is a second and extremely important matter. In fact, this may be the most important aspect

Exhibit 6-1 Four Principal Phases of PPO Development

Phase	Major Characteristics
1. Feasibility	● Define objectives of PPO development.
	● Undertake feasibility study to determine if these objectives can be achieved. Feasibility components:
	a. Legal
	b. Marketing
	c. Provider relations
	d. Financial
2. Planning	● Refine feasibility estimates, particularly market penetration and impact on financial operations.
	● Construct work program for initial PPO development operations.
	● Important issues: Provider selection criteria, payment methods for physicians and hospitals, discount levels, utilization controls, incentive systems for physicians, data system requirements.
3. Development	● Establish legal entity: PPO.
	● Draft and sign contracts: providers, purchasers, and subcontractors (e.g., for utilization review or claims administration).
	● Implement data system for utilization review, program monitoring, management decision making.
	● Begin marketing to primary groups.
4. Operational	● Provide medical services.
	● Market to new groups.
	● Begin monitoring impact of PPO on length of stay, charges, etc.

of the feasibility study, for without physicians and hospitals, there is no preferred provider arrangement.

An understanding and an analysis of individual markets and the marketability of the PPO concept in the community represent the third component of the feasibility study. Certain conditions suggest a readiness of major purchasers to link themselves with preferred provider arrangements. High levels of employee cost sharing are indicative of purchaser interest in PPOs. Conversely, where major employers typically pay 100 percent of employee claims, incentives for employees to use preferred arrangements will be limited. The marketability of a preferred provider organization in such an environment would face difficult, if not insurmountable, obstacles.

The preferred provider organization feasibility study culminates in a projection of whether or not the PPO will produce revenue that exceeds the costs of operation, and determination of the sources of this revenue. The financial portion of the feasibility study will also consider the financial impact of the preferred provider organization on individual providers, namely, acute care hospitals when the PPO is hospital sponsored. The four components of a PPO feasibility study are examined in the following chapters.

Chapter 7

Assessing Markets and Purchaser Interest

At a fundamental level, marketing success is highly contingent on knowledge of the relative needs and wants that specific groups may have for the product being made available to them. The ability to tailor the product to individual groups serves as an important indicator of future accomplishment and success.

The marketing feasibility phase is characterized by the collection and analysis of data on purchaser groups expected to purchase the product of the preferred provider organization.

PRIMARY MARKETS AND CONSUMER NEEDS

Preferred provider arrangements established in the early 1980s placed an emphasis on marketing to self-funded, or self-insured groups. In metropolitan areas like Denver, Colorado, labor union trust funds and self-funded employers became the principal markets for developing preferred provider organizations. Arrangements developed subsequently have also leaned on these two particular markets. There is, however, a growing recognition that a preferred provider organization can reduce the cost of its marketing program by "piggybacking" its services onto the products and services of organizations such as third party administrators and employee benefits brokers, which themselves have significant clientele.

From the perspective of the emerging preferred provider organization, the principal market segments are employee benefits programs, third party administrators, self-funded corporations, labor union trust funds, insurance companies, and, eventually, the individual subscriber. Exhibit 7-1 identifies some of the particular needs that each of these market segments may have.

Some third party administrators (*all* should) view preferred provider organizations as an important tool for maintaining and increasing their client base, i.e., those organizations for which they perform claims administration activities.

Exhibit 7-1 Major PPO Market Segments

Market Segment	Needs
Third party administrator	• Control rising claims for corporate and labor clients
	• Increase client base due to cost containment success
Employee benefits brokers and consultants	• Keep current clients by linking them into cost-efficient delivery systems
	• Acquire new clients because of linkages
Insurance carriers	• Control premium increases so current groups do not shift to other carriers or become self-funded
	• Reduce total volume of claims paid, resulting in greater profit margin
Self-funded employers and unions	• Control claims/premiums
	• Control hospital utilization
	• Administrative simplicity
	• Minimize labor problems as the result of implementing benefit changes
	• Ensure high-quality care for employees
	• Ensure that the PPO will not go bankrupt
Subscribers	• Limit out-of-pocket payments
	• Choice of physicians and hospitals
	• Convenience: geographic and time-related

One can speculate that third party administrators have an interest in controlling medical claims for their clients only to the extent that their clients have voiced a concern about rising claims experiences. Third party administrators with some vision realize that the ability to control medical claims experiences will be linked directly with their ability to maintain and expand claims administration, their primary business.

The concept of "piggybacking" applies to employee benefit brokers and consultants as well as third party administrators. Major national and international brokers/consultants have a sizable reservoir of corporate clients who seek ongoing consultation and advice from them. Again, the brokers/consultants have a primary interest in retaining current clients and acquiring new ones by linking them into cost-efficient delivery systems.

The needs of self-funded employers and labor union trust funds are more oriented to the issue of controlling medical claims. It is in the direct financial interest of these groups to exercise some element of control over the magnitude of medical care claims. These organizations have also indicated a very clear intent to control hospital utilization, since hospital utilization is closely associated with the magnitude of the claims experience.

A third need is for administrative simplicity. Those organizations large enough to be self-funded or self-insured face all of the bureaucracy and corporate problems of any large corporation or organization. The ability of an employee benefits manager or vice-president of personnel to quickly enter into a contractual relationship with a preferred provider organization is associated with the administrative simplicity of that arrangement. If the preferred provider organization requires self-funded organizations to utilize a new claims administration agent or if other substantial changes are required, perhaps in the employee benefit package, the administrative simplicity disappears. In this environment, one can expect the corporation or labor trust fund to respond in slow fashion.

These organizations also have an interest in the quality of care provided to employees by the preferred provider organization. Poor-quality services reflect on the employer or trust fund, and may ultimately produce labor problems. Thus, the avoidance of labor problems can be defined as an additional and salient need of these particular market segments. Finally, large self-funded employers and labor union trust funds will be particularly concerned about the stability of the preferred provider organization. In the late 1970s and early 1980s, a number of health maintenance organizations went through bankruptcy proceedings, creating administrative and management problems for those purchasers that had made the health maintenance organizations available to their employees. These purchasers have no interest in repeating this experience.

Insurance carriers have two primary goals. The first, like that of the third party administrator and employee benefits brokers/consultants, is to control premium increases so that the insurance carrier can maintain its subscriber base. Persistent yearly premium increases of a sizable nature provide an impetus for subscriber groups to seek other carriers and/or pursue the route of self-funding. In addition, insurance carriers, because of their profit motive, have an economic need to reduce the total volume of claims paid, producing a greater profit margin for the insurance company.

The subscriber, too, has certain needs that must be met by preferred provider arrangements. Subscribers are interested in limiting or eliminating out-of-pocket payments. Under appropriate conditions, preferred provider organizations can meet this need. Subscribers also have an interest in choosing the physicians and hospitals from which they receive their care. This does not necessitate that subscribers have an unlimited ability to select any health care provider but, rather, suggests that a wide choice should be available. The size of that choice will affect the attractiveness of the preferred panel. Convenience is a perceived need mentioned frequently by the consumer market. Preferred provider organizations offering a limited geographic distribution of providers or a panel of providers that is beyond the travel preference of the subscriber population will face marketing difficulties.

These five groups, then, represent the major segments of the preferred provider organization market. As for future market segments, there is every reason to believe that both state and federal governments will eventually provide economic incentives for Medicaid recipients and Medicare patients to seek care from preferred panels of medical care providers. California's Selected Provider Contracting Program and Arizona's AHCCCS program are two state efforts designed to channel Medicaid recipients into cost-efficient groupings of health care providers. Federal government demonstration programs to include Medicare enrollees in health maintenance organizations suggest that this population will have access to preferred panels in the future. Developing preferred provider organizations will want to consider these two large populations as PPOs evolve.

MARKET FEASIBILITY TASKS

Market feasibility assessment is a process of systematically analyzing the extent to which individual companies, union trusts, and other purchasers are willing to participate in a preferred panel arrangement. The output of the market feasibility process is the determination of (1) the individual purchasers most likely to participate and (2) the level of services they will purchase through the PPO. The former provides information critical to the marketing function of the PPO. The latter can be an important indication of the influence the purchasers may have on participating providers, particularly hospitals.

The market feasibility outputs involved require a general understanding of three interrelated concepts: the gross market, the service area, and primary market groups. The gross market can be characterized as the total number and distribution of individual purchasers the PPO initially believes to have an interest in its product. In its most elementary form the gross market is a listing of purchasers meeting broadly defined criteria. These criteria typically include the size of the purchaser, its location, and a subjective assessment about the seriousness of the purchaser's interest in cost control. Once the gross market has been plotted, it is necessary to identify the distribution of employees or union members associated with the groups comprising the market. Informal interaction with individual companies or with brokers/consultants can provide a general understanding of where employees may live. Without the direct involvement of companies and brokers/consultants in this process, it will be necessary to make rough estimates in this area.

A second marketing task is the delineation of the preferred provider organization service area. The service area of a preferred provider organization is that geographic area in which the majority of panel providers, purchasers, and subscribers are located. In general, its size is determined by the farthest distance that a subscriber/patient is willing to travel to receive care from a preferred provider. Therefore, it is usually identical or highly similar to the geographic distribution of the gross market. Some purchasers located on the periphery of the service area, such as a larger company, may employ many persons who reside a substantial distance away. In such cases, the PPO may wish to either expand its service area by adding providers located in proximity to those populations or to eliminate those populations from its initial marketing efforts.

In defining the service area, it is mandatory that some standard be established for geographical access. Studies suggest that consumers will probably not travel beyond a maximum of 20 or 30 minutes for medical care except in rural environments. The service area must be generally consistent with the distribution of physicians, hospitals, pharmacies, and other health-related groups linked to the preferred provider organization.

In a practical sense, the distribution of the major market segments should serve as a force eventually determining the distribution of the providers. For example, if a PPO were to geographically plot both its potential subscriber population and providers linked with the PPO, and find a major geographical discrepancy between the two, the expansion and increased distribution of the providers would appear to be a more appealing alternative than the truncation of the service area.

A third market feasibility task is the acquisition and analysis of demographic data on the defined service area population. It should be recognized that the characteristics of the service area population may or may not be the same as the characteristics of the purchasers comprising the gross market. Though the demographic analysis may be inexact, it can be helpful in providing certain types of information. Age and sex information will help the preferred provider organization determine whether an adequate number of certain physician specialties are in the immediate area. A community having large numbers of young children and/or women of child-bearing age will indicate an obvious need to ensure that the PPO panel includes an adequate number and distribution of pediatricians and obstetrician/gynecologists who practice in that area. General information on the population density will also help the preferred provider organization ensure that the ratio of physicians to population is adequate to treat the medical needs of the particular area.

The last major task of the market feasibility study is the collection and analysis of detailed information on primary market groups. The primary market is a subset of the gross market. It is composed of individual purchaser groups exhibiting the greatest potential for involvement in the PPO. The identification of primary market groups is accomplished by surveying all of the purchasers included in the gross market. The results of the survey provide the basis for eliminating low-priority groups from the initial marketing of the program. For example, a PPO may have identified 30 sizable purchasers as being its gross market. On closer examination, however, the PPO may find that only 20 of these have large enough populations residing within the service area to warrant the immediate attention and effort of the preferred provider organization. The initial 30 companies represent the gross market; the primary market becomes the 20 with populations located in the confines of the service area.

The determination of the primary market groups, however, is dependent on far more than the mere geographical location of subscribers' employees or union members. If certain purchasers pay 100 percent of all medical claims and cannot reduce their payment level, it is highly unlikely that those purchasers would find a preferred provider organization attractive. Such purchasers are unable to offer incentives for employee/patients to limit themselves to a select number of physicians and hospitals when their health benefits pay 100 percent for the use of any hospital or any physician. An important determinant of a primary market group, then, is the existence of employee cost sharing, primarily at the 80 percent level.

Primary market groups are also defined by the management attitude within the group. Large corporations that have articulated an extremely strong interest in cost containment and are willing to pursue innovative cost-containment programs are also far more likely to be good candidates for a marketing program.

The cosmopolitan nature and the age structure of a purchaser group also helps determine which groups will comprise the primary market. Young, cosmopolitan (employee) groups are less likely to have lengthy, established relationships with particular health care providers. These groups can be expected to be more liberal in the choice of their physicians and hospitals, and be more inclined to use preferred provider organizations when they are available.

Exhibit 7-2 provides a generic format for collecting data on potential subscriber groups. The recommended format identifies the level of cost sharing; it also attempts to collect information on residence patterns, employer attitudes towards the PPO, changes that may be necessary to accommodate the PPO, and the primary hospitals used by employees, union members, or subscribers. Primary hospitals are also identified so that the PPO can assess the extent to which it may wish to expand hospital participation. If very large groups are using a small number of hospitals, it may be valuable to seriously consider including those hospitals in the preferred provider organization if mutually agreeable contracts can be reached.

An outgrowth of the survey will be information on potential PPO use. Table 7-1 contains estimates of the number of persons likely to use the preferred panel and the practical implications this has for the PPO in terms of ambulatory and hospital utilization. Note that preferred panel use rates are tied closely to incentive levels: the greater the level of employee/patient cost sharing, the greater the PPO

Exhibit 7-2 An Example of a Format for Collecting Data on Potential
Subscriber Groups

General Information

Name of group: Hapless Enterprises
Address: 11111 Avenue Boulevard
Telephone: 100-582-4134
Employee benefits manager: W. G. Hilliard

Health Insurance or Coverage Information

Number of employees covered: 15,500
Number of dependents covered: 35,000
Insurance carrier: Self funded; uses B.H.M. Administrator
Services covered and payment arrangements:
  All inpatient and outpatient services covered except inpatient alcoholism treatment
  Deductible:
    $100 individual
    $200 family
  Copayment
    80% up to maximum of $2,000 including deductible
Expiration date: Not applicable

Group Residence Patterns

Estimated percent of employees/dependents residing in specific communities:

Community	%
Medford	80%
City View	5%
Oxmond	5%
Heathertown	5%

Employer Attitude Toward PPOs:

Do key purchaser executives (V.P. personnel, finance or employee benefits) favor PPO participation?
  Yes . . . though tempered by concerns noted below
Are they willing to make internal changes necessary to accommodate PPO participation, on a timely basis?
  Yes, but they are concerned about their ability to integrate PPO provisions into the labor management contract which does not terminate for 10 more months. This contract covers all benefit agreements between labor and management.
Does the purchaser have specific requirements which the PPO must meet?
  V.P. Personnel refuses to change third party administrator. PPO must accommodate this arrangement if their business is desired. Also the Chief Financial Officer (CFO) wants a semi-annual statistical report quantifying cost savings, and has indicated that the company will not pay more than 1.5% (of total claims) as an "access fee" to the PPO.

Hospital Utilization

Number of hospital days used per 1,000 employee/dependents (most recent year):
  658 patient days per 1,000 covered

Exhibit 7-2 continued

Primary hospitals used:
  Doctors' Hospital
  Nurses' Hospital
  R. Blackmore Memorial Hospital

use rate. As noted earlier, operational preferred provider arrangements have exhibited use rates of 50 to 80 percent when patients face copayments of 20 percent or more for use of nonpanel providers. Physician and hospital utilization data are not necessarily a marketing issue. However, they should be generated from surveys of purchaser groups because they aid at least two other feasibility components. Such information allows a developing PPO to more accurately gauge the size and distribution of the provider based needed to adequately care for the estimated patient pool. An excess of providers dilutes the effect that the PPO will have on individual physicians and hospitals. Having too few providers opens the door to short-term customers and eventually long-term marketing problems.

The patient volume information also assesses financial feasibility analyses, in particular that financial component which examines the relationship among (1) hospital discounts, (2) the level of increase in inpatient volume needed to effect discounts, and (3) the influence of these on the revenue base of individual participating acute care institutions.

PURCHASER PARTICIPATION

Purchaser participation in preferred panel arrangements is contingent on several matters including (1) the ability of the PPO to demonstrate probable purchaser savings, (2) internal labor-management relationships, and (3) internal corporate legal advice about PPO-related liability. This statement highlights a difficulty reported consistently by developing PPOs. That is, major purchasers have been slow to formally commit to PPO involvement, for the above reasons, even though these same purchasers have been vocally aggressive in their statements about medical care cost containment.[1]

It becomes imperative, then, that emerging PPOs give serious consideration to these matters in the feasibility process. A community-based coalition in western Michigan conducted a PPO feasibility study during the first half of 1984. Their work provides insight into the manner in which feasibility studies might address major purchaser concerns.[2]

Table 7-1 Estimating Patient Volume, by Purchaser Group

Purchaser Groups	Total Number of Employees/ Dependents To Be Offered PPO	Current Cost Sharing Provisions (Family Coverage)	Financial Incentives/ Decentives Planned To Stimulate PPO Usage	Estimated Number of Persons To Regularly Use Preferred Panel	Rationale	Estimated Number of Physician Visits At 6 Visits Per Person Per Year	Estimated Number of Hospital Days at 750 Days Per 1,000 Persons
Big Tire International	5,000	• $200 deductible • $100 maximum out-of-pocket • 90% paid by employer	• No deductible • No out-of-pocket • 100% paid	15% (450 persons)	Limited penetration due to low employee cost sharing	2,700 visits	338 days
Buford Agri-Business	5,000	• $500 deductible • $2,000 maximum out-of-pocket • 80% paid by employer	• No deductible • 100% paid	35% (1,250 persons)	Significant positive incentive to use preferred panel	7,500 visits	938 days
International Brotherhood of Computer Programmers	1,000	• No deductible • $500 maximum out-of-pocket • 100% paid by trust fund	• No out-of-pocket	Less than 5% (50 persons)	Lack of cost sharing; users will be those currently using preferred panel	300 visits	38 days

Table 7-1 continued

Purchaser Groups	Total Number of Employees/ Dependents To Be Offered PPO	Current Cost Sharing Provisions (Family Coverage)	Financial Incentives/ Decentives Planned To Stimulate PPO Usage	Estimated Number of Persons To Regularly Use Preferred Panel	Rationale	Estimated Number of Physician Visits At 6 Visits Per Person Per Year	Estimated Number of Hospital Days at 750 Days Per 1,000 Persons
Auto-Rite Bodyworks, Ltd.	10,000	• No deductible • $2,000 maximum out-of-pocket • 80% paid by employer	• 50% paid if preferred panel *not* used	50% plus (5,000 persons)	Significant disincentives if preferred panel not used	30,000 visits	3,750 days
State Medicaid Program	15,000	• No deductible • No out-of-pocket • 100% paid by state	Previously uncovered preventive services available when PPO panel is used	Less than 5% (540 persons)	Lack of cost sharing; users will be those currently using preferred panel	2,700 visits	338 days
TOTAL	36,000	N/A	N/A	7,200	N/A	43,200 visits	5,402 days

Estimating Purchaser Savings

The western Michigan PPO feasibility study concluded that participating purchasers would financially benefit from PPO association for five reasons:

1. The PPO would include a small number of high-quality, yet low-cost facilities. Persons participating in a PPO would be directed to these efficient institutions rather than a broad spectrum of facilities, many of which are several hundred dollars more costly per admission.
2. Further, persons using nonparticipating facilities would, in most circumstances, assume greater financial responsibilities for the cost of such care.
3. Hospital utilization would be reduced.
4. Additional cost savings could be generated by discounts offered when a predefined volume of medical services had been reached.
5. Premium increases could be expected to be less for insured companies. Those moving to self-funding and PPO participation could expect sizable reductions.

In estimating the financial impact on any given purchaser, certain assumptions must be made. For the purposes of the western Michigan study, the following assumptions were used:

- Company size: 100 employees/350 persons insured
- Insurance: Self-funded with stop-loss
- Ratio of hospital expenses to total health expenses: 60%
- Employee coverage:
    $100 deductible per employee
    Hospital costs: 80% paid by company
    Physician and other medical services: 80% paid by company
- Hospital utilization:
    600 pt. days/1,000 persons per year
    90 admissions/1,000 persons per year
- Adjusted average cost of PPO-affiliated hospitals: $2,245 per admission (1982 information)
- Adjusted average cost of non-PPO hospitals: $2,637 per admission (1982 information)
- PPO incentive structure:
    If PPO providers are used, employee coverage remains as above.
    If non-PPO providers are used, coverage changes:
        $100 deductible per employee
        60% of hospital services paid by company

60% of physicians and other medical services paid by company
- Panel use rate: 80% (80% of persons used preferred physicians and hospitals)
- Current hospital use preferences:
  50% use PPO-affiliated hospitals
  50% use non-PPO-affiliated hospitals
- Discounts: 10% (based on volume minimum)
- Expected impact of utilization review: 6% net reduction in costs due primarily to reductions in number of admissions

Impact Due to Incorporation of Cost-Efficient Hospitals

The above assumptions suggest that prior to PPO participation, 50 percent of the example company's covered persons would have used non-PPO hospitals while the remaining 50 percent would have already been using those facilities eventually associated with the PPO program. The total cost of hospital care with this split would have equaled $61,513. After the availability of the PPO program, however, the feasibility study estimated 80 percent of all covered persons would use PPO participating facilities while 20 percent would continue using non-PPO participating providers. This panel use rate (80 percent) is consistent with PPO experiences in other locations. The change in use patterns would have resulted directly from the PPO incentive structure (see assumption). The cost of hospital care in the latter case would have totaled $55,227. This estimate of savings resulted from the difference in hospital costs before and after PPO participation and, further, from reduced company payments (60 percent versus 80 percent), which would have occurred for those persons who would have elected to continue to use nonparticipating facilities.

In the western Michigan study, the difference in hospital costs ($6,286) equaled a 10.2 percent reduction in the cost of hospital services or a 6.1 percent savings in the total costs of care, because hospital-related costs were estimated to be 60 percent of total corporate health expenditures.

Cost Savings Due to Utilization Reductions

The western Michigan study assumed a conservative estimate of a 6 percent reduction in the rate of admissions for that 80 percent of employees/dependents eventually using PPO providers. The study considered this to be a new reduction figure, which means that it also accounted for any outpatient services resulting from the reduced admission rate. The net reduction of 6 percent produced an additional hospital savings of $2,716 (4.4 percent) from the pre-PPO figure of $61,513. This equaled a net savings of 2.6 percent in the total corporate health costs. Again, hospital costs were assumed to represent only 60 percent of total corporate health expenditures.

Cost Savings Due to Self-Funding

The exact benefits a company would receive from self-funding would depend on many factors. The western Michigan PPO study concluded that an additional 10 percent savings could be expected by companies currently insured that pursue the advantages of self-funding.

Discounts

Some PPOs initiate discounts with hospitals and physicians, others don't. For the purposes of assessing purchaser cost-containment benefits, the western Michigan study assumed that no discount would be offered by either hospitals or physicians until a certain level of PPO volume had been reached. Volume-based discounts were considered to represent a unique situation in which slight economies of scale (experienced by providers because of their preferred status) could be passed on to purchasers.

The study assumed that a 10 percent discount would be offered by both physicians and hospitals, but this discount level would apply only to 75 percent of total services purchased; that is, the first 25 percent of services purchased represented the period of no discounts, the critical volume necessary before discounting was considered appropriate.

A 10 percent volume-based discount on hospital services was found to produce a 3.6 percent net savings in total corporate expenditures. A similar volume-based discount on physician services produced a 2.4 percent net savings.

Based on the assumptions and conditions specific to the western Michigan PPO feasibility study, it was determined that self-funded companies could expect to experience a 14.7 percent cost savings; companies that went from traditional insurance to self-funding were expected to see even larger savings (see Table 7-2).

The western Michigan assessment applied these savings to a multiyear model. Most of the companies considering PPO participation were small. Accordingly, the multiyear projection of cost savings was based on a company with 1984 annual health claims (or premiums) of $250,000. Table 7-3 contains the study's estimates of savings, over time, resulting from PPO participation.

The simple model used in the western Michigan study provided potential purchasers with a realistic estimate of the tangible benefits they could expect if subsequent PPO participation materialized.

Table 7-2 Estimated Cost Savings, as a Percent of Total Company Health Expenditures by Source

Source	Percent Savings
Incorporation of Efficient Hospitals	6.1%
Utilization Reductions	2.6%
Self-Funding	10.0%
Volume Discounts on Hospital Services (at 10% on 75% of Services)	3.6%
Volume Discounts on Physician Services (at 10% on 75% of Services)	2.4%
	TOTAL:
For Self-Funded Company	14.7%
For Company Becoming Self-Funded	24.7%

Table 7-3 PPO Cost Savings, Illustrated for Companies with Annual Health Claims/Premiums of $250,000

	1984	1985 (10% inflation)	1986 (10% inflation)	1987 (10% inflation)
Self-Funded Company, with PPO Participation	—	234,575	258,033	283,836
Without PPO Participation	250,000	175,000	302,500	332,750
Annual savings	—	40,425	44,467	48,914
Newly Self-Funded Corporation with PPO Participation	—	207,075	227,783	250,561
Traditional Insurance Coverage without PPO Participation	250,000	275,000	302,500	332,750
Annual Savings	—	67,925	74,717	82,189

Internal Labor Management Relationships

A group that plays a crucial role in the marketing success of an emerging PPO is organized labor. Corporations may have a strong interest in PPO affiliation. If, however, they are not able to constructively work with organized labor to initiate internal benefit changes allowing this to occur, participation will not occur. It is in the direct interest of new preferred panel programs to understand the perspective of labor groups and the forces that determine how they feel about preferred provider programs.

The western Michigan feasibility study provides an insight into these matters. That study, after interacting with labor, came to the following conclusions:

> The economic realities of the 1980s have been difficult for organized labor. Wages and benefit levels have been held constant or reduced in a variety of industries. Employee groups have also assumed more financial responsibility for benefits, notably, health care. Employee financial participation in premium payment, deductions and general co-payment have been common.
>
> Even though labor has slowly assumed increasing financial obligations for health benefits, leading one to expect that interest in cost control programs would be considerable, predictable concerns exist about doing this.
>
> First, labor's experience with the benefit reductions of prior years makes interim contract negotiations concerning benefit changes immediately unappealing. [The study] . . . initiated early interaction with labor. The principal purpose was to determine if labor would be willing to open interim contract negotiations with management, allowing necessary incentives to be incorporated into health benefit packages so that employees could be financially rewarded for prudent buying behavior, i.e., using PPO providers. Interaction with labor has led to the following conclusions on labor/management relations:
>
> - Some labor bargaining units would be favorably inclined to discuss benefit changes with management. This willingness would be a direct reflection of overall labor/management relations in a particular company.
> - If labor were to give up certain items, such as limiting choice . . . that is, current benefits would only be provided when a PPO provider was used . . . labor would expect to share in the cost savings generated by their actions.
> - The major labor group is the AFL-CIO affiliated Allied Industrial Workers (AIW). This group represents about 70% of organized labor and many AIW contracts will undergo scheduled negotiation in 1986. It is clearly to the advantage of these groups to begin discussions with management now, rather than to wait for the pressure of overall negotiations. There can be no doubt that health benefits will be a central issue of scheduled negotiations; early

discussions offer the potential for fully examining the magnitude of rising medical expenditures and, most importantly, finding acceptable solutions which meet the needs of both labor and management.

A second fundamental concern of labor is comprehensiveness of services. A PPO would be attractive only to the extent that it has broad provider participation and is able to incorporate a full range of services. This perspective closely mirrors critical areas of interest articulated by business.

A related matter concerns labor's stated interest in Health Maintenance Organizations. HMOs offer comprehensive services frequently requiring no or very little direct payment on the part of an employee or his/her family. A preferred provider organization would need to closely parallel HMO (1) comprehensiveness and (2) absence of employee out-of-pocket costs, if it were to be found appealing to the labor community.[3]

Preferred provider programs, like the Greater Baltimore PPO, have recognized the need to interact with labor early in the marketing process. The absence of such interaction nationally has led to a general slowness on the part of select purchasers to participate in PPOs. There can be no doubt that aggressive PPOs will increasingly give early attention to labor management problems that have the potential to handicap market development.

GENERAL INDICATORS OF MARKET FEASIBILITY

In the final analysis, the market feasibility study must incorporate value judgments and subjective considerations, along with the data gathered in this phase of feasibility assessment. General indicators that may be supportive of the preferred provider organization include the following:

- Positive attitude on the part of large employer/employee groups as well as employee benefits brokers and consultants.
- The ability of participating hospitals to care for the projected load of patients generated through the preferred provider organization.
- Increasing levels of copayment within the community; frequent labor troubles associated with contract negotiations resulting from efforts by management to increase employee cost sharing may be indicative of increasing efforts to expand employee financial participation in health benefits.

- A close association between the anticipated distribution of physicians and hospitals and primary market groups.
- In general, an employee copayment level of about 20 percent or greater throughout major market segments.

PURCHASER INFORMATION REQUIREMENTS

Regardless of sponsorship, preferred provider organizations require information capabilities that allow five key activities to be performed.[4] Initially, a PPO entity should have quantitative data for the selection of efficient, competent physicians and hospitals. Second, at an ongoing level, information describing the efficiency with which medical services are delivered must be monitored. Third, physicians ideally need immediate feedback on the efficiency of their individual practice patterns. Fourth, PPO clients (purchasers) must be routinely informed about the benefits and savings derived from participation. Finally, and most obvious, a PPO must track a variety of quality, cost, revenue, and activity trends for itself and for provider participants.

Most of these management data requirements have been covered in other sections, with the exception of the data requirements necessary to attract and keep purchaser involvement. Tables 7-4 through 7-6 provide examples of minimal data purchasers should receive from PPO involvement. Table 7-4 provides a summary of both benefits paid during the reporting period and the direction of that payment. This table gives a purchaser an understanding of the amount of care purchased in different settings: hospital care, outpatient hospital services, emergency care, physicians' services, nursing and home health care, and other benefits. Noncovered charges as well as deductibles and adjustments are also highlighted in this report.

A particularly useful aspect of the benefits expenditure report is that column displaying the percent of payment directed toward the individual settings in which care was received. The example shows that the majority of expenditures in the reporting period were for inpatient and outpatient hospital care, with substantial payments for physician services associated with hospital-based medical treatment. A comparison of these percentages over time assists a purchaser in assessing whether the preferred provider organization is effectively shifting the focus of care from an inpatient to an outpatient setting. In fact, if this is occurring, the percent of payments for hospital care should decline and, conversely, payments to physicians for outpatient services as well as for outpatient hospital services should increase. The reporting format suggests further that this information be compared with similar financial information for those individuals not using the select panel of health providers. Again, an examination of the percent

Table 7-4 An Example: Health Benefit Expenditures, by Category for Third Quarter, 1983

Type of Care Provided	Expenditures for PPO Patients	% of Total PPO Expenditures	Expenditures for non-PPO Patients	% of Total Expenditures for non-PPO Patients
Inpatient Hospital Care	$42,000	42%	$96,000	48%
Outpatient Hospital Care	14,000	14%	20,000	10%
Emergency Services	8,000	8%	24,000	12%
Physician Services Provided in Hospital	12,000	12%	28,000	14%
Physician Services Provided in Office	6,000	6%	10,000	5%
Nursing Home Care	3,000	3%	2,000	1%
Home Health Care	5,000	5%	—	0%
Pharmacy and Other	10,000	10%	20,000	10%
TOTAL	$100,000	100%	$200,000	100%

Table 7-5 Example of Utilization and Charge Information by Diagnostic Grouping for Third Quarter, 1983, PPO Participants

Diagnostically Related Group	Number of Admissions	Total Days	Average Length of Stay	Average Charge	Total Charges for Reporting Period	Total Charges Year to Date
DRG 39: Lens Procedures	100	300	3.0	$1,650	$165,000	450,000
DRG 373: Normal Delivery Without Complications	100	370	3.7	2,500	250,000	692,000
DRG 294: Diabetes, age 36 and above	10	70	7.0	2,100	21,000	59,000
DRG 088: Chronic Obstructive Pulmonary Disease	30	300	10.0	3,200	96,000	407,000
DRG 127: Heart Failure and Shock	50	600	12.0	6,300	315,000	1,010,000
DRG 243: Medical Back Problems	20	200	10.0	3,300	66,000	198,000
TOTAL	310	1,840	5.9	2,944.9	913,000	2,816,000

Table 7-6 Comparative Utilization and Charge Information by Diagnosis, PPO Use Versus Non-PPO Use, Third Quarter, 1983

Diagnostically Related Group	Average Length of Stay	Average Charge	Average Length of Stay	Average Charge	Difference in Charge Per Admission	× Number of PPO Admissions	= Net Savings
DRG 39: Lens Procedures	3.0	$1,650	3.5	$1,820	$170	100	$17,000
DRG 373: Normal Delivery	3.7	2,500	3.6	2,600	100	100	10,000
DRG 294: Diabetes, Age 36 and above	7.0	2,100	7.6	2,430	340	10	3,400
DRG 088: Chronic Obstructive Pulmonary Disease	10.0	3,200	9.5	3,000	(200)	30	(6,000)
DRG 127: Heart Failure and Shock	12.0	6,300	11.7	6,300	0	50	0
DRG 243: Medical Back Problems	10.0	3,300	12.5	3,950	650	20	13,000
TOTAL							$37,400

of payments directed toward individual settings of care will aid the purchaser in assessing the overall efficiency orientation of the PPO.

All other things being equal, one would expect (hope) to find that the percent of payments to preferred providers would be less for in-hospital care than that paid for those individuals not using the select panel. This assumption is based on the existence of effective utilization controls employed in the PPO arrangement.

Further, purchasers need adequate information on major diagnostic categories and the charges for those categories for both PPO participants and those not using the PPO panel. Table 7-5 displays the minimum generic data a purchaser should expect from a preferred provider organization: number of admissions for the reporting period, average length of stay, total charges, cumulative payments per DRG for the reporting year and for the year to date. Diagnostically specific information is desired because it provides a common denominator for purchaser assessment. While individual diagnoses or diagnostically related groups are preferred, larger groupings of data are useful when diagnosis-specific information cannot be obtained. In such instances, diagnostic categories (obstetrics, circulatory disorders, digestive disorders, lymphatic and blood diseases, etc.) can be used to provide admittedly rough comparisons from one reporting period to the next, and between PPO participants and non-PPO users.

Table 7-6 is a variation of the above reporting format. Individual diagnostic categories or procedures are compared on the basis of average length of stay and total charges for PPO and non-PPO patients. The purpose of this comparison is to provide the purchaser with a periodic report on cost savings generated for the most costly aspect of medical programs: hospital services. Similar tables might be established for ambulatory procedures. By comparing the frequency and charges associated with common costly ambulatory services an additional understanding of cost savings can be realized.

NOTES

1. Carol Cain, "Wisconsin Employers Not Sure About PPOs," *Business Insurance* (May 12, 1984): 31; "Investor-Owned Hospitals Study PPO Concept: Leaders of Industry Adopt 'Wait and See' Policy," *F.A.H. Review* 15, no. 4 (July/August 1982): 40–42; *Meidinger, Inc., Health Care Cost Containment Survey* (Pittsburgh: Meidinger, Pittsburgh, October 1983); *Meidinger, Inc., Health Care Cost Containment Survey* (Cincinnati/Dayton/Columbus: Meidinger, Cincinnati, October 1983).

2. S. Brian Barger and David G. Hillman, *Preferred Provider Organizations and Grand Haven Michigan: A Feasibility Assessment* (Cincinnati, Oh.: Morgan Bigae Institute, June 1984).

3. Ibid.

4. Sallie J. Drury, "Employers Pick PPO Data Over Discounts," *Business Insurance* (March 12, 1984): 25.

Chapter 8

The Health Care Provider: Assessing the Feasibility of Participation

In determining the probability of eventual participation of health providers in a preferred provider organization, one issue is prominent: does sufficient interest, cooperation, and commitment exist among an adequate number of physicians and hospitals with a geographically dispersed pattern of services to make the preferred provider program attractive to prospective purchasers? The provider participation feasibility component is perhaps the most subjective and least quantitative of the feasibility components discussed. Assessing cooperation and interest are inexact arts ultimately based on subjective evaluation by those conducting the feasibility study.[1]

Before discussing critical aspects of provider participation feasibility, it should be mentioned that there are certain environmental indicators that point to the willingness of physicians and hospitals to ally themselves with PPOs. If an excess number of hospital beds exist in a community and if hospital occupancy rates are substantially below 80 percent, hospitals, in all probability, will be exploring a variety of mechanisms for increasing their patient volumes. When there is a surplus of physicians, and when private practice physicians observe patient waiting times for appointments dwindling from two weeks to two days, physician concern about future patient volume is also heightened. Hospital occupancy rates, excess beds, appointment waiting times, and physician-to-population ratios are quick and easy tools for assessing whether the health care provider community will embrace and participate in preferred arrangements.

PHYSICIAN INVOLVEMENT

Typically, evolving preferred provider arrangements have strong ideas about which institutions they wish to serve as the focal point of acute care for their program. Assessing physician interest in PPO activities, then, most naturally starts with the medical staff of the identified institutions.

In highly competitive environments characterized by excess physician populations, written communications may serve as one mechanism for identifying
physician interest. In most cases, however, informal communication such as that
done on a personal basis, will provide a much less threatening environment in
which to discuss possible physician PPO involvement. When, in aggregate,
physicians perceive a threat from competing physicians, recognize the need to
change consistent with pressures of cost containment, and understand the generic
benefits of PPOs, the assessment may be that broad-based physician involvement
is probable.

The informal discussion phase of the physician participation feasibility study
also serves to identify key, established physician leaders. These leaders, once
they have a full appreciation for, and interest in, PPO activity, can serve as
liaisons with the remainder of the respective medical staff. The ability to identify
and involve the established physician leaders is critical. The inability to do so
will produce difficulties for any PPO wishing to enroll a sizable portion of a
given hospital's medical staff.

The physician participation feasibility component also explores the willingness
of medical practitioners to accept competitive fee structures, participation requirements, utilization review procedures of a vigorous nature, and the ongoing
collection of information that may be used to gauge physician efficiency.

Physician cooperation is one of the most important though intangible ingredients of the PPO feasibility. Such cooperation does not imply acquiescence to
the whims and policies of the legal PPO entity, whether it be provider, purchaser,
or investor sponsored. Rather, it suggests physicians' willingness and commitment to constructively participate in and, indeed, debate the design and implementation of those aspects of the organization that are likely to affect them.
Moreover, cooperation implies compromise. Preferred provider arrangements,
like Kansas City's Mid-America Health Network, involve multiple hospitals and
medical staffs; they must balance numerous competing values and interests for
the viability of the organization.

The breadth of specialty participation in the PPO must also be studied. Does
it appear that an adequate number of obstetrician-gynecologists, radiologists,
surgeons, neurologists, and other specialties are prepared to participate? Con-
tingency plans need to be implemented in those particular situations where a
small number of specialty physicians enroll in the medical panel. Having only
a small number of specialty practitioners will eventually lead to long waiting
periods for those services, and will adversely influence the reputation of the
preferred provider arrangement.

The PPO physician participation assessment must further consider geographic
distribution of providers. By graphically plotting the distribution of interested
physicians within high-priority communities, the PPO can begin to determine
the appropriateness of physician distribution. The graphic comparison of the

physician population to the potential subscriber population also helps to pinpoint potential problems. Rapidly growing or larger areas with a very limited number of panel physicians, or areas with a large number of children but a very low number of participating pediatricians, are examples of potential trouble spots.

A final aspect of the physician participation feasibility component concerns the willingness of practitioners to accept the unique arrangements. Aetna Life and Casualty has initiated a PPO-type program called Choice, in both the Chicago and Washington, D.C., areas. These programs allow virtually any primary care practitioner to participate; however, participating practitioners must agree to refer all patients only to a very limited number of hospitals and the specialty physicians on the medical staffs of those hospitals.[2] If similar type structures are envisioned for developing preferred provider organizations, the willingness of physicians to accept these unique arrangements must be considered.

ASSESSING HOSPITAL PARTICIPATION

The assessment of hospital involvement in preferred provider organizations parallels that discussed for physicians.

One of the most important aspects of the hospital assessment concerns institutional efficiency. When available, assessment of diagnosis-specific information, including comparison of it with that of other institutions or norms, is highly desirable. Such comparisons should focus on the average charge per admission and average length of stay for high-frequency diagnoses. Other general methods for selecting efficient hospitals were covered earlier in Chapter 7.

The hospital assessment, like that for physicians, should consider the willingness of individual facilities to accept (1) discounts, (2) unique payment mechanisms (per diem or per case), and (3) aggressive utilization review activities, in particular, preadmission certification.

The existence in a community of an appropriate mix of participating facilities that consider religious and other preferences of the population to be served should also be examined. A PPO using a limited number of Protestant-affiliated hospitals, for example, may have serious difficulties in marketing its program to communities that are largely Jewish or Catholic. These preferences may intensify for selected services such as obstetrics.

The financial stability of providers, particularly institutions, is another important area for consideration. Hospitals with significant levels of debt, or those unable to operate efficiently, run the risk of facing severe financial difficulties in the future. A PPO must determine whether it wishes to associate with these facilities. The reputation of hospitals that may participate in the preferred panel of providers is the last item of consideration. A preferred provider organization enhances its marketability when it includes low-cost, high-quality, efficient institutions that have established solid reputations. At best, involvement with facilities of questionable reputation may slow the growth of the preferred provider organization; at worst, it may serve as a factor that eventually brings on the demise of the PPO.

The provider participation assessment discussed here has not addressed the matter of other providers: pharmacy, skilled nursing, home health care, etc. Preferred provider arrangements should consider contractual arrangements with these providers. Certain PPOs, such as Aetna's Choice and John Deere's corporate-sponsored organization, have entered into mutually advantageous contracts with local pharmaceutical chains, skilled nursing facilities, and home health care agencies. These services should be available to purchaser participants; a PPO's attractiveness increases as it integrates other such services at significant discount levels or through highly competitive fee structures.

NOTES

1. For additional perspectives on provider participation see S.J. Tibbits and A.J. Manzano, *Preferred Provider Organizations: An Executive's Guide* (Chicago: Pluribus Press, 1983), 47–59; Health Service Policy Group (AMA), *A Physician's Guide to Preferred Provider Organizations* (Chicago: American Medical Association, 1983), 57–78.

2. " 'Choice' Health Plan May Hamper Care, D.C. Physicians Warn," *American Medical News* (September 9, 1983): 1+.

Chapter 9

Financial Issues in PPO Assessment and Development

The financial phase of a feasibility assessment addresses two primary issues. First, a major consideration is the source of revenues that will be used to operate the PPO entity and the extent to which these revenues equal the costs of operation. These matters are of immediate interest to the PPO entity, which may or may not be associated with a particular hospital. Second, from the standpoint of an individual hospital, financial feasibility relates directly to the association between (1) discounts that the facility may offer to the PPO and (2) the degree to which the hospital, through its association with the PPO, will experience the positive financial benefits resulting from increased patient volume. An individual hospital will consider PPO association financially feasible when the revenue generated by increased business offsets competitive fee arrangements offered to attract such business.

In the remaining portion of this chapter, financial feasibility is examined both from the orientation of a PPO entity and from that of an individual hospital considering PPO participation.

COSTS ASSOCIATED WITH THE PLANNING AND DEVELOPMENT OF PPOs

The newness of preferred provider organizations and the speed with which many have been established accounts for the general lack of information on developmental and planning costs. The identification of planning and development costs is further hampered by the developmental path many preferred provider organizations have taken. That is, PPOs have been created by individual hospitals or groups of physicians that provide substantial amounts of manpower, resources, and technical services (data systems) of an in-kind, rather than cash, nature.

Planning and development expenditures fall in four principal areas: (1) legal fees, (2) marketing programs and materials, (3) staffing and personnel costs, and (4) costs associated with computer hardware and software for management information and utilization monitoring activities.

Legal services can be substantial and costly. (Chapter 10 will address legal and regulatory concerns in depth.) Preferred panel arrangements frequently require the establishment of a new corporation and concomitant development of articles of incorporation and corporate bylaws. Contracts must be drafted for physicians, hospitals, pharmacies, nursing homes, home care services, utilization review bodies, and purchasers. Other legal services may also be desired. Newly formed PPOs may, for example, require legal consultation concerning the structure of the corporation to avoid potential antitrust problems. Legal assistance sought in testing a PPO's structure against Federal Trade Commission or U.S. Justice Department standards can also result in further legal expenses. Health Care Management Associates in New Jersey and Hospital Corporation of America are two organizations that have received wide publicity for their efforts to acquire advisory opinions.

Marketing programs require advertising and a variety of materials. General descriptive materials must be developed for providers and purchasers interested in affiliation. Once these groups become formally associated other marketing and program materials need to be prepared, such as

1. A physician's handbook detailing PPO procedures, policies, and operational guidelines
2. Consumer marketing materials: physician/hospital inventories, program summaries, benefit comparisons

Personnel costs are the direct result of the staff required to plan and initially develop a preferred panel arrangement. Independence Medical Systems, of Clearwater, Florida, for example, used about two full-time equivalent professionals to initiate its program. Mid-America Health Network in Kansas City relied heavily on one key hospital staff member, as did Penrose Hospital's PPO program in Colorado Springs, Colorado, and ScrippsCare, the PPO program affiliated with Scripps Memorial Hospital in San Diego, California. Other PPOs have reported similar initial staff patterns using 1 to 2.5 professionals.

Personnel costs are also a function of the length of time required to adequately plan and develop a program. Tulsa's CompMed worked for an estimated 60 days to establish its program. The pace of this developmental effort was driven by the outgrowth of expanding competition from developing prepaid medical systems. But such short time frameworks are uncommon. ''Day One'' of actual operation is typically preceded by 9 to 18 months of planning and development.

The costs of computer hardware and software can be expected to vary widely depending on the scope and needs of an individual preferred provider program. Consumer Medical Cost Containment Corporation has developed a sophisticated, computerized software package for utilization control and monitoring, the cost of which is estimated at $150,000. Others, like Actuarial Associates of America, have microcomputer programs available for $40,000–$60,000.

The cash value of total planning and developmental costs for the four major expenditure areas reviewed above are estimated to be between $175,000 and $300,000. This estimate range is drawn from three PPO programs (Ohio, Michigan, and Florida), which reported estimated preoperational costs including personnel/consultant, marketing, legal, and data software expenses.

OPERATIONAL COSTS AND REVENUE SOURCES

There are several ways that the operating cost structure of a preferred provider organization might be defined. For the purposes of a feasibility assessment component, PPO operating costs refer specifically to management, marketing data, and utilization review activities. This does not encompass all of the possible expenditures associated with a preferred provider organization: hospital care, physician care, etc. The reason for not including these costs is simple. As an entity, the preferred provider organization is not at risk for the costs of hospital or physician care; these costs are borne directly by individual purchasers. The preferred provider entity, though, is financially at risk for the costs of its own operation. The critical issue to be considered by the feasibility assessment planner is whether or not adequate revenue can be obtained from a variety of sources to cover the administrative, marketing, data, and utilization review costs.

Several potential revenue sources are available; the PPO must assess which are the most feasible to tap.

1. Participating hospitals may contribute directly to hospital-sponsored PPOs; because many preferred provider organizations have been established as tax exempt, nonprofit organizations by individual facilities, these facilities can and have effectively donated in-kind services and resources to the PPO entity.
2. Another source of revenue being used increasingly is the physician participation fee. The fee may be as little as $25 per year, or it may approach $1,000 per year, the fee employed by the Physicians' Alliance for Medical Excellence. Such a fee is large enough to underwrite the costs of a PPO's operation.

3. A hospital participation fee or management fee may be levied. Hospitals in California's Universal Health Network, for example, pay a monthly fee of $2,500 for the marketing management and other services of the network.
4. For-profit joint venture PPOs may use annual equity contributions from participants to meet expenses. Scripps Memorial Hospital Healthcare Management System, a for-profit joint venture between the hospital and members of its medical staff, uses such a system.
5. Purchasers may pay an access fee for having the opportunity to use the preferred panel and the competitive fee structures negotiated by the PPO. Access fees in the range of 1–2 percent of total claims by purchasers have been reported. These fees are typically translated into a monthly charge per employee/subscriber.

At the present time there is little consensus on whether or not an "access fee" should be charged to participating subscriber groups. Parenthetically, it should be noted that a "Catch-22" situation appears to be developing with the concept of an access fee. Proprietary PPOs, by their very nature, typically need to charge some type of fee to purchasers so that adequate revenue can be generated to underwrite overall operating costs. Provider-sponsored PPOs have not necessarily felt the economic need to charge the access fee. From a provider perspective, financial gains come from increased utilization and market share, not from profits generated, per se, from the purchaser sector. As a result, provider-sponsored preferred provider organizations typically do not require an access fee from purchasers. The obligation of the purchaser is to provide an agreed-upon economic incentive to employees, encouraging them to seek PPO services. This produces a dilemma for proprietary preferred provider organizations as well as for multiple PPOs in a single community. One can assume that purchasers will participate in the lowest-cost, highest-quality preferred provider organization. All things being equal, provider-sponsored programs have a clear advantage in this regard.

Preferred provider organizations may subcontract the claims administration function or they may interact with a variety of claims administration agents, depending on which agents are used by individual subscribing groups. Regardless of which method is used, it is common for the preferred provider organization to divorce itself from the costs of claims administration; that is, the purchaser interacts directly with the claims administrator and pays the claims administration fee directly to the third party administrator. This approach minimizes the administrative burden on the PPO and allows it to accommodate a wide variety of claims administration agents.

Utilization review is conducted in equally diverse ways. Hospital-sponsored PPOs may merely use their existing internal review programs to monitor care rendered to PPO subscribers. Frequently, though, a PPO subcontracts this function to a qualified review body like a foundation for medical care or a designated peer review organization. The costs of the review program may be assumed by the PPO and passed on to the purchaser, assumed directly by the purchaser, or, infrequently, borne by the PPO (usually hospital based).

LINKING REVENUES TO EXPENDITURES

Defining annual operating costs for a PPO is a highly inexact art at this point in PPO evolution. Annual operating budgets from existing preferred arrangements do, however, facilitate this process. Such budgets serve as a very rough approximation of the operational expenses a mid-sized PPO might expect. Two PPOs, one in the South, the other in the West, have reported annual operating budgets of slightly less than $120,000. One of these involves about 120 physicians; the other twice that.

In the remainder of this section the annual expenses that a PPO might face will be estimated and options will be presented for generating the revenue to underwrite these expenses and, possibly, produce an operating margin or profit. Table 9-1 outlines the various assumptions used in this example.

ESTIMATING TOTAL ANNUAL OPERATING COSTS

Total annual operating expenses for the PPO are composed of amortized development costs, base annual operating expenses, and the cost of subcontracted utilization review services. In our example we will assume that the PPO entity wishes to recover and pay to the "lenders" the $175,000 invested in the de-

---

Table 9-1 PPO Costs, Revenue and Utilization Assumptions

---

a.	PPO Development (Pre-Operational) Costs:	$175,000
b.	Base Annual Operating Expenses	$120,000
c.	Initial PPO Subscriber Base	250,000 covered persons
d.	Preferred Panel Use Rate	50%
e.	Historic Hospital Use Rate of Subscriber Base	500 patient days per 1,000 persons
		100 admissions per 1,000 persons
f.	Utilization Review Cost per Admission	$40 per admission
g.	Number of Participating Providers	3 hospitals
		500 physicians
h.	Total Claims Paid by Purchaser	$100,000,000

velopment of the program. Assuming this figure, with interest, totals $200,000 and that this payback occurs over a 5-year period, $40,000 must be added to the base operating expenses. Our example also assumes that the PPO will incur the costs of utilization review, for which it has subcontracted with an appropriate review body at a negotiated fee of $40 per admission (which covers preadmission certification, concurrent length of stay review, and retrospective studies). The first year annual cost of this service can be projected as follows:

$$\frac{\text{Annual Utilization}}{\text{Review Costs}} = \text{ISB} \times \text{PPUR} \times \text{AR} \times \$$$

where:

ISB	=	Initial subscriber base
PPUR	=	Preferred panel and use rate
AR	=	Admission rate
$	=	Review cost (per admission)

Using the example presented in Table 9-1, an estimate of the costs would be as follows:

$$\text{Annual review costs} = 250,000 \times .50 \times \frac{100}{1,000} \times \$40$$

$$= \$500,000$$

The total annual operating costs of the PPO, then, would be $660,000.

Identifying Sources and Levels of Revenue

Our example assumes that the PPO entity has decided to recover its total operating expenses for the three principal beneficiaries of the program: physicians, hospitals, and purchasers. Further, the organization has determined that it must generate an adequate annual operating margin/profit, which it has set at 10 percent. Accordingly, a margin of $66,000 has been added by the PPO to expenses, producing a total revenue need of at least $726,000.

The PPO could decide to acquire all of its revenue from the purchaser. This could be accomplished by charging a flat fee either for each covered person (250,000) or for each patient admission (12,500) resulting from the use of the preferred panel. Each of these methods would produce purchasers' access fees of $2.90 per covered person or $58.08 per admission.

But other options are available. Table 9-2 illustrates four options that a PPO might pursue to meet or exceed its revenue needs.

Options A and D are particularly consistent with the structure of hospital-sponsored nonprofit programs. Hospital management and physician participation fees paid to the PPO entity are not excessive; the purchaser fees of $500,000, regardless of how these are calculated, merely coincide with the estimated utilization review cost normally assumed by purchasers. Option C more closely parallels a hospital-sponsored for-profit PPO, or a for-profit joint venture between hospitals and physicians. The reasons for this are twofold. First, the hospital management fee is $109,000 per institution, a very substantial amount. Such levels of investment are usually associated with for-profit ventures in which the amounts paid are actually equity contributions rather than management fees. Also, the purchaser access fee fails to meet the normal expenses of review. This implies that the PPO is far more interested in the beneficial impact it has on

Table 9-2 Revenue Sources and Various Options for Meeting/ Exceeding PPO Revenue Needs: An Example

Basic Revenue Sources	Options			
	A	B	C	D
Purchaser Access Fee Equal To:*				
● ¼%			$250,000	
● ½%	$500,000			
● 1%		$1,000,000		
Purchaser Fee Equal To Cost or Review Only	—	—	—	$500,000
Physician Participation Fee (per Physician)**	@$200 = $100,000	$0	@$300 = $150,000	@$300 = $150,000
Hospital Management Fee (per Hospital)	@$42,000 = $126,000	$0	@$109,000 = $327,000	@$26,000 = $78,000
Total Revenue Generated per Year	$726,000	$1,000,000	$727,000	$728,000

*Percent of total claims paid ($100,000,000)
**In for-profit PPOs, these may be equity contributions.

provider participants (volume increases, market share enhancement) than the actual profitability of the PPO entity. Under such circumstances provider sponsorship seems most likely.

The large cash profit produced by purchasers in option C readily suggests an entrepreneurial base. Access fees, in general, are a reflection of proprietary PPOs. This is indicated further by the absence of any fees for physicians and hospitals, a condition designed to attract significant provider participation and, accordingly, contribute to the PPO's market appeal.

PPO financial feasibility can and must extend beyond the simple yet helpful parameters explored here. For hospital-sponsored programs, concerns will be (1) the extent to which discounts affect the revenue position of participating institutions and (2) the level of increased volume necessary to offset varying levels of discounts. These and related matters are explored in the following section.

INSTITUTIONAL FINANCIAL FEASIBILITY

The most basic goals of all PPO participants are the fundamental economic precepts of minimizing losses and maximizing revenue. These underlying principles are the common denominator of all financial feasibility assessment. That is to say, then, that institutional assessment of the financial feasibility of PPO participation is not significantly different from that performed by individual providers or purchasers. The method of analysis and variables may differ to some degree, but all feasibility assessments include two basic elements: some projection of volume of service units to be provided or purchased and the cost of providing or purchasing those units of care. For a hospital, the critical elements become (1) the number of patient days attributable to PPO participation, (2) the relationship of those days to total patient days provided, (3) the number of current non-PPO days converted to PPO patient days, (4) revenue generated by both PPO and non-PPO days, and (5) the cost of providing any and all days of care. In sum, the issue becomes one of assessing whether, within the context of PPO participation, a hospital's total revenue will be equal to or greater than the total cost of providing care. More simply said, a hospital wants to know if it is going to lose money by participating in a PPO.

Basic Considerations

Prior to assessing the impact of participation upon its revenue there are two basic considerations to be made. First, if a hospital is considering PPO sponsorship, it will need to determine the "startup" or development cost. As was discussed, the capital outlays for development can be hefty, ranging from $175,000 to $300,000 in some cases. On the other hand, if an existing PPO approaches a hospital with an invitation to participate, the hospital's only real "startup" cost may be an initial "participation fee." These are generally not prohibitive. Second, if a hospital wishes to sponsor a PPO, it must consider the source and amount of funds required to underwrite the administrative functioning of the PPO. These may take the form of an equity contribution, an in-kind contribution, or a variety of other arrangements. These may be substantial, especially if marketing and administrative programs are elaborate, or if legal problems arise.

Components of Revenue Impact Analysis

When the basic organizational and operational cost issues have been addressed, the hospital may proceed with an analysis of impact upon revenue. Four major components may be identified. They are (1) volume of service, (2) cost, (3) revenue, and (4) a payment mechanism. A fifth component, case-mix intensity, is an important one and should be considered in a financial feasibility analysis. It is, however, of relative importance to volume and revenue and not, in fact, a major component of financial feasibility evaluation.

Since there is most likely no PPO experience upon which to draw, projections of the volume of patient days attributed to PPO participation must necessarily be based on historical patterns of utilization, accounting for expected future environmental change. Ideally, projections should be made with the highest degree of accuracy possible and a range should be calculated whose minimum and maximum parameters permit a variety of activity and alternative action plans. Projections of new PPO days, non-PPO days, non-PPO days converted to PPO days, and total patient days will be needed.

When projections of patient days have been made, the cost of the delivery of those days may be estimated. Because a range of volumes has been projected, it will be necessary to consider the effect of various utilization levels on individual cost behavior patterns. There are four individual cost components that comprise an institution's total cost. Each of the four behaves in a different fashion from the others, varying (or not) with volume, dependent upon the nature of the cost. The individual elements of total cost are (1) fixed cost, (2) semifixed cost, (3) variable cost, and (4) semivariable cost.

Fixed costs are those that remain constant regardless of changes in volume of service. Semifixed costs tend to behave in similar fashion, exhibiting a flat curve until critical volumes are reached. At those critical volumes, the entire cost curve shifts to a higher level. Variable costs are those that vary in direct proportion to volume. Semivariable costs, like variable costs, vary in direct proportion to volume but will experience a shift in the cost curve as critical volumes are reached.

Semifixed and semivariable costs are subsets of fixed and variable costs, respectively, and are available only in the most sophisticated of settings. Most analyses will include fixed and variable cost components alone.

Once an anticipated volume range has been established and cost components identified, the two remaining financial elements, payment mechanism and revenue, may be considered. The fee structure established must generate sufficient revenue to cover the projected total cost, which includes (1) capital expenditures, (2) an allowance for return on equity (for investor-owned facilities) and/or operating margin, and (3) an amount to cover discounts (i.e., Medicare, Medicaid, Workmen's Compensation, Blue Cross, etc.) and bad debts. The amount of revenue necessary to cover discounts and bad debts will vary considerably among institutions, with a normal range being approximately 10 to 16 percent. The levels of discounts and bad debts in the projection must be analyzed with the same intensity as cost. Projections must include any anticipated change in the patient and case (diagnosis) mixes historically maintained. Changes in patient mix will alter the third party payment source and, because of varying reimbursement agreements, will change projected revenue and, in some cases, cost reimbursement. Economic conditions such as increases in unemployment will have an impact on bad debts.

Alternative Rate Structures

A number of rate and/or charge structures may be utilized by institutions participating in a preferred provider organization. However, in considering any reimbursement arrangement it should be kept in mind that any rate established which is less than that now being paid will decrease revenue unless there is a positive change in patient mix or volume.

The degree of sophistication of current data on utilization and cost may continue to dictate the type of reimbursement arrangements that are feasible or may, at a minimum, indicate the degree of risk involved in participation. Payment mechanisms currently utilized, in order of popularity, include (see Table 9-3):

- Percent of billed charges (discounts)
- Per diem payment
- Diagnosis Related Group (DRG)-based payment
- Incremental cost-based payment

The most popular payment mechanism is a method that permits the consumer or, in actuality, the purchaser, to pay a percent of total billed charges. The reasons for the popularity of discounting billed charges are simplicity and the ability of the provider to predict the financial impact of participation. This method

Table 9-3 PPO Payment Mechanisms: Advantages and Disadvantages

Reimbursement Types	Method of Payment	Advantages	Disadvantages
Discount off Total Billed Charges (May be Service Specific)	Percent of Total Billed Charges	Ease of Understanding Ease of Calculation Predictability of Financial Impact (Limited Risk Which is Reduced Further on Service Specific Agreements Inclusion of Non-Patient Care Cost (i.e., Teaching and Research)	Decreases Net Revenue as a Percent of Gross Revenue (Assuming No Volume Change) Establishes Necessity for Cost Shifting if Volume Does Not Increase
Per Diem (may be Service Specific)	Fixed Payment For Each Day of Confinement	Ease of Understanding Ease of Calculation Predictability of Revenue Based on Change in Patient Days (Assuming No Case Mix Change) Inclusion on Non-Patient Care Cost	Decreases Net Revenue as a Percent of Gross Revenue (Assuming No Volume Change) Establishes Necessity for Cost Shifting if Volume Does Not Increase Increases Risk of Negative Financial Impact if Volume Increases in High Cost Service Areas Requires More Comprehensive vs. Data Systems to Monitor Case Mix

Table 9-3 continued

Reimbursement Types	Method of Payment	Advantages	Disadvantages
Diagnosis Related Group (DRG)	Fixed Payment Per Case Based on Diagnosis (May be Percent of Previously Established DRGs)	Reduces Risk of Negative Financial Impact Due to Change in Case Mix Increases the Relationship Between Revenue and Specific Service Cost	Requires Increased Knowledge of Costs Related to Diagnosis Payment May be Negotiated to Exclude Non-Patient Care Functions (If Percent of DRG is Utilized Cost Shifting Will be Necessary Without an Increase in Volume) Possible Negative Medical Staff Reaction Due to Pressure for Reduced Length of Stay
Incremental Cost	Fixed Payment For Individually Identified Cost Centers (May be Per Diem Supplemented by Special Services)	Increases Relationship Between Revenue and Specific Service Cost Reduces Risk of Negative Financial Impact Due to Change in Case Mix	Requires Increased Knowledge of Costs Related to Specific Service Components Payment Negotiated to Exclude Non-Patient Care Cost

can be applied on a service-specific basis, i.e., medical/surgical, obstetric, pediatric, psychiatric, or other. Discounts also produce immediate savings for purchasers and are, therefore, often an excellent marketing tool for providers. The per diem charge is also easy to calculate and understand; however, the determination of financial impact necessitates a thorough knowledge of the current case mix and accurate predictions of changes in case mix. This method may also be applied on a service-specific basis.

The Diagnosis Related Group (DRG)-based payment, currently being implemented by the federal government for Medicare patients, is now being viewed as an alternative payment mechanism by other purchasers. This method of prospective payment eschews hospitals' charges for individual services or products, such as patient days, x-rays, laboratory tests, etc., in favor of payment for aggregated service per case. Case-mix management then becomes a vital element in future financial analysis. However, to be effective, case-mix management must include detailed cost budgeting for the various diagnosis categories. Current management information systems have, in most cases, not yet obtained the level of sophistication necessary to adequately project the impact of the use of a DRG-based payment mechanism. The popularity of DRGs as a payment mechanism should increase as the currently limited experience is expanded and as information systems become more sophisticated and reliable.

Payment based on incremental cost has limited applicability at the current time. The necessary determination of detailed cost figures for each service element, i.e., room and board, operating room, etc., is, in most institutions, simply not possible. Furthermore, this method requires additional negotiation time dependent on the number of services for which rates are individually determined. For an institution offering thousands of services, both the time and cost of developing these systems are prohibitive.

The payment mechanism selected and the rate structure (as well as its relation to cost) will, for the most part, depend on the ability of the institution to define its cost and case mix, and will depend further on its perception of its ability to maintain or increase its market share.

A MODEL FOR PPO FINANCIAL FEASIBILITY ASSESSMENT

The model described below can be a simple, effective method used by an institution in assessing the probable financial impact of PPO participation. The model is designed to produce for an institution projections of PPO revenue, non-PPO revenue, and PPO patient days required for the hospital to break even with, or exceed, current net revenue levels. It requires only a minimum of simple, readily available information and utilizes uncomplicated step-by-step calculations. Furthermore, the model can be expanded, as necessary or desired, to accommodate a greater variety of more complex information, e.g., semifixed and semivariable costs.

The model is based on two assumptions about the future that relate to its workability. The first assumption is that there will be no change in the volume of patient days in the short run (first year). In essence, the hospital is treating a full year's data as a cross-section, i.e., as a single point in time. This is required since the model is static, rather than dynamic. Second, the hospital assumes that all PPO days will be paid for, that is, no bad debt or other deductions (except the discount) will be incurred from PPO days. Since PPO enrollees are most often insured by carriers and self-funded employers, the assumption is more than reasonably valid.

The only prerequisite to the operation of the model is the collection of basic information that will be used as, or used to calculate, variables that input the model. The basic information required by the model includes

- number of beds
- estimated occupancy rate
- average charge per day
- percent of total deductions from revenue
- estimated total cost
- percent of total cost that is fixed cost
- percent of total cost that is variable cost

All other inputs to the formula may be derived from these.

When the basic information has been gathered, the model may be implemented. The four basic steps, as detailed below, are (1) calculation of input variables, (2) calculation of PPO revenue/cost, (3) calculation of non-PPO revenue/cost, and (4) calculation of the number of PPO patient days required for the hospital to recover its discount. The illustration assumes that the payment mechanism is a discount from billed charges.

Step 1: Calculate Input Variables

The calculated variables that input the model are:

1. Projected patient days = (beds × 365 days per year × occupancy rate)
2. Gross revenue = (patient days × average charge per day)
3. Deductions from revenue = (gross revenue × percent deductions from revenue)
4. Net revenue = (gross revenue − deductions from revenue)
5. Net revenue per day = (net revenue/patient days)

6. Cost per day = (total cost/patient days)
7. Fixed cost per day = (cost per day × percent fixed cost)
8. Variable cost per day = (cost per day − fixed cost per day)

It is likely that the hospital will have projected patient days prior to operating the model, in that methods used to compute the basic information (total cost, etc.) require the patient days variable. If so, that calculation may be unnecessary. Note, however, in examining the list of variables and formulae, that none except projected patient days may be calculated solely from the basic information. Calculation of each of the rest is dependent on one or more of the inputs whose calculation preceded it. Accurate calculation is critical. One small miscalculation may be compounded into gross error, resulting in financial feasibility being greatly misstated.

At this point, the hospital must arbitrarily estimate the expected number of patient days that will be attributable to PPO enrollees. These are subtracted from projected total patient days to yield non-PPO patient days. The resulting PPO/non-PPO dichotomy is the basis for Steps 2 and 3. (Recall the suggestion to calculate for a range of patient day volume. To facilitate illustration, however, a range is not calculated here. Note further that all four major components of financial feasibility assessment discussed earlier are now present. Again, they are service unit, i.e., patient days, cost, revenue, and payment mechanism.)

Step 2: Calculate PPO Revenue/Cost

The six elements of the PPO revenue/cost component are:

9. Total billed PPO billed charges = (PPO days × average charge per day)
10. Discount from PPO billed charges = (PPO billed charges × discount rate)
11. PPO revenue = (PPO billed charges − discount)
12. PPO revenue per day = (PPO revenue/PPO days)
6. Cost per day = (as calculated in Step 1)
13. PPO net revenue per day = (PPO revenue per day − cost per day)

The calculation of PPO revenue/cost figures is not difficult. Projected total PPO billed charges, based on the number of PPO patient days previously estimated, are discounted by the specified rate to produce a projection of revenue attributed to PPO utilization. The PPO revenue is then divided by the number of PPO days, yielding net revenue per PPO day. Cost per day, which was calculated in Step 1 by dividing total cost by total patient days, is subtracted from PPO net revenue per day to determine the net contribution of revenue over cost per PPO patient day. It is here that the first indicator of the financial feasibility of participation appears. If the difference between revenue and cost is not positive, the institution will lose money by participating in the PPO. It may also suffer losses if the difference is positive; however, that situation is determined only after the operation of Step 3.

Step 3: Calculate Non-PPO Revenue/Cost

The elements of the non-PPO component are:

14. Non-PPO revenue = (net revenue − total PPO billed charges)
15. Non-PPO revenue per day = (non-PPO revenue/non-PPO days)
 6. Cost per day = (as calculated in Step 1)
16. Non-PPO net revenue per day = (non-PPO revenue per day − cost per day)

The calculation of non-PPO elements mirrors that of the PPO element illustrated in Step 2. The obvious exception is that the calculation of a discount is unnecessary. Non-PPO revenue is divided by non-PPO days, thus calculating non-PPO revenue per day. Cost per day is then subtracted from that figure to find the daily net revenue provided by non-PPO days. The resulting difference will be a positive number (unless the institution operates at a loss) equal to the operating margin that has been built into the charge/revenue structure.

The level of non-PPO net revenue per day determines break even, which is the minimum level of PPO net revenue per day that is required for PPO participation to be financially feasible for the hospital. As stated in the description for Step 2, PPO net revenue per day may be a positive number, yet the hospital may find itself at a financial disadvantage by participating in the PPO. Participation is not financially feasible if the amount of PPO net revenue per day is greater than zero, but falls short of the non-PPO net revenue per day. The hospital may or may not necessarily incur a loss at the bottom line; however, its operating margin, or profit, will be eroded by the smaller amounts of PPO revenue accrued. This may require an increase in the average charge per day to compensate for the lost operating margin—that is, if the institution chooses to participate.

It is no coincidence that the maximum percent discount that can be offered to a PPO by a provider is equal to the percent of deductions from revenue. Any percent discount greater than the percent of deductions from revenue will produce a PPO net revenue per day that is less than the non-PPO net revenue and, therefore, the institution's revenue will decrease. A rule of thumb, then, is that an institution's percent of deductions from revenue represents the maximum discount from billed charges that it can offer PPO participating purchasers without losing revenue.

Step 4: Calculate PPO Patient Days Required To Recover Discount

The subcomponents of PPO discount recovery are:

12. PPO revenue per day = (as calculated in Step 2)
8. Variable cost per day = (as calculated in Step 1)
17. PPO net revenue per excess day = (PPO revenue per day − variable cost per day)
18. PPO patient days required to recover discount = (discount from PPO billed charges/PPO net revenue per excess day)

Assuming that an institution's fixed costs are paid for by the estimated total number of patient days (both PPO and non-PPO), any additional PPO day will generate excess revenue that is equal to PPO net revenue per day less the variable cost per day. Said differently, that excess revenue is equal to the fixed cost per day calculated in Step 1, plus the PPO revenue surplus per day calculated in Step 2. The number of PPO days over and above those originally projected that will cause recovery of the discount is determined by dividing the PPO net revenue per excess day into the discount from PPO billed charges that was calculated in Step 1. Furthermore, once the discount has been recovered, each additional PPO day generated adds dollars to the institution's net revenue in an amount equal to PPO net revenue per excess day. Needless to say, these excess days most often add large amounts to the hospital's bottom line.

A SIMPLE APPLICATION OF THE MODEL

The following review illustrates an application of the generic model outlined above and should help to clarify any uncertainties.

Consider a scenario wherein a hospital has been invited to participate in a PPO, beginning January 1, 1985, and has been asked to offer participating purchasers an 11 percent discount from its billed charges. Assume further that the hospital, in its strategic planning, has made some estimates for 1985 and that it predicts that 1,200 of its total patient days will be accounted for by the PPO.

Basic Information:

- Number of beds: 350
- Estimated occupancy: 78%
- Average charge per day: $425

- % Deductions from revenue: 14.2%
- Total cost: $35,608,838
- % Fixed cost: 40%
- % Variable cost: 60%

Step 1: Calculate Input Variables

1. Projected patient days: 99,645 (350 × 365 × .78)
2. Gross revenue: $42,439,125 (99,645 × 425)
3. Deductions from revenue: $6,013,576 (42,439,125 × .142)
4. Net revenue: $36,335,549 (42,439,125 − 6,013,576)
5. Net revenue per day: $364.65 (36,335,549/99,645)
6. Cost per day: $357.36 (35,608,838/99,645)
7. Fixed cost per day: $142.94 (357.36 × .40)
8. Variable cost per day: $214.42 (357.36 − 142.94)

Step 2: Calculate PPO Revenue/Cost

9. Total PPO billed charges	$510,000
10. Discount from PPO billed charges	$56,100
11. PPO revenue	$453,900
12. PPO revenue per day	$378.25
6. Cost per day	$357.36
13. PPO net revenue per day	$20.89

Step 3: Calculate Non-PPO Revenue/Cost

14. Non-PPO revenue	$35,825,549
15. Non-PPO revenue per day	$363.91
6. Cost per day	$357.36
16. Non-PPO net revenue per day	$6.55

Step 4: Calculate PPO Patient Days Required To Recover Discount

12. PPO revenue per day	$378.25
8. Variable cost per day	$214.42
17. PPO net revenue per excess day	$163.83
18. PPO patient days required to recover discount	343

Among the several important pieces of information available to the hospital at this point are:

- A PPO patient day generates $14.34 more revenue per day than a non-PPO day. The reason is that the PPO discount (11 percent) is smaller than the percent of deductions from revenue (14.2 percent). (Compare items 13 and 16.)
- Item 17 indicates that each PPO patient day in excess of the 1,200 originally estimated will produce $163.83 in additional revenue. (Add items 7 and 13.)
- Item 18 shows the hospital that if the 1,200 PPO days originally estimated are exceeded by 343, then the hospital will have recovered its discount (item 10) on the 1,200 days. In essence, provision of 1,543 PPO patient days effectively converts 1,200 patient days to full pay ($425 per day). If the institution does not participate and adds 1,543 patient days it will be paid only $363.91 for each. In sum, the hospital will add $78,226.62 more revenue to its bottom line if it participates in the PPO, and 1,543 PPO patient days are delivered, than if it does not participate.

The discount rate in this example is based on charges, not cost. This does not preclude consideration of cost as a base from which to work; however, the discount should be taken from existing billed charges.

The general formula for calculating the increase in patient day volume necessary to compensate for a discount from billed charges is:

$$I = \frac{(p)(c)(d)}{r - v}$$

where

I = Number of PPO days required to recover discount
p = Estimated number of PPO days
c = Average daily charge
r = PPO revenue per day
v = Variable cost per day
d = Discount rate

In the scenario presented above the calculation would appear as:

$$I = \frac{(1200)(425)(.11)}{378.25 - 214.42}$$
$$I = \frac{56,100}{163.81}$$
$$I = 343$$

Though this analysis was presented from the viewpoint of an institution, consideration by individual practitioners assessing participation in PPOs is not significantly different in concept. The payment mechanism must include consideration of charges, revenue, and cost to calculate the financial impact of PPO participation.

The payment mechanism utilized depends on the philosophy of the PPO and, to some degree, acceptance by the individual provider. The most common payment mechanisms at the current time are (1) discounted usual, customary, and reasonable charges (UCR) and (2) a predetermined dollar amount applied to a relative value scale (RVS) for each defined procedure. The decision an individual practitioner must make is similar to that made by an institution. Obviously, the amount of net revenue required by an individual varies with the financial requirements and/or goals of the individual. That is to say that the individual, like the institution, wishes to minimize patient loss, maintain current patient volume, or increase patient volume.

While a financial impact analysis of PPO participation is essential, there are other factors related to financial decision making that must be considered.

FURTHER FINANCIAL FEASIBILITY CONSIDERATIONS

The development of, or participation in, a PPO may, in the short run, alter several factors used to evaluate financial feasibility. The two most important factors are (1) a change in volume and (2) a change in the patient and/or case mix.

Anticipation of a positive change in volume is, in most cases, the reason for agreeing to participate. Once the volume level increases to a point to permit recovery of any rate differential, all additional increases in the short run add to total revenue. The higher the ratio of fixed cost to total costs, the more each additional unit will add to revenue. However, some PPOs are requesting variable rates based on volume. As volume increases, the ratio decreases in prescribed increments. As an example, the PPO and institution may agree upon a rate of 90 percent of billed charges for an estimated patient volume of 5,000 PPO days, the rate to be reduced to 88 percent if total days exceed 10,000.

Any agreement of this type requires a more sophisticated analysis to determine financial impact. As discussed earlier, in the short run there are semifixed costs that will increase as patient volume reaches defined levels. The cost of some administrative services are examples of semifixed costs. As we saw earlier, it is necessary to increase personnel in some areas as certain volume levels are reached and exceeded. Semivariable costs behave in similar fashion. Regulations requiring specific staffing ratios related to patient volume fuel semivariable cost increases. The sophistication necessary to predict variable rate impact requires the addition of semifixed and semivariable cost functions to the model.

An increase in volume, in most cases, can be considered a positive aspect of PPO participation. However, an increase can be negative if the payment mechanism does not account for changes in patient and/or case mix. If the method of payment is a per diem charge, or to a lesser extent, a discount from total billed charges, and does not consider service-specific categories or diagnoses, a change in case mix from low-cost to high-cost services will have a negative impact on revenue. It is essential that, at a minimum, cost be defined on a service-specific basis to reduce risk. Also, the more closely charges reflect cost in all areas, the lower the risk under any rate payment method. The prospective payment system based on diagnosis related groups (DRGs) currently being implemented by Medicare will expedite cost/service relationship analysis.

A consideration that should be made in any assessment of PPO participation is impact on cash flow. Reducing the age of accounts receivable from an average of 45 days to 14 days allows for lower reimbursement levels, if desired. The reduction of accounts receivable by 30 days based on a per diem revenue of $375 would mean, at 8.5 percent interest, $2,655 per month in additional revenue for 1,000 days of care. Any increase in cash flow should be considered to offset any discount in the negotiated rate when analyzing PPO participation.

An important factor for consideration, in the long run, is a change in the scale of operations. The capital investment necessary to accommodate a change in the scale of operations must be carefully weighed. Capital expenditures increase total fixed costs, which, in turn, increase not only the cost per day, but also the ratio of fixed to variable cost. This statement is made on the assumption that volume does not increase. If volume increases, the cost increase and relationship of fixed to variable cost may or may not increase, depending on the magnitude of the capital expenditure and the extent of volume increase.

The decision to increase the scale of operation must be carefully considered. If an increase in volume results in a decrease in unit cost, net revenue will increase. The reverse is also true. If unit cost is increased, net revenue will decrease. However, if the payment rate is based on diagnosis, capital expenditure may or may not affect the revenue/cost relationship. That will depend on the allocation of cost to specific services and the existing case mix. The same is true if the payment rate is based on incremental cost. It is vital that the cost of new capital expenditure be allocated to the particular service to which it applies if the impact is to be appropriately analyzed.

The institutional analysis of financial feasibility of PPO participation is not necessarily a difficult or costly process. It may most definitely be tailored to the needs and budgets of the individual institution. It may be simple or sophisticated, gross or detailed. Clearly, what it must not be, however, is overlooked.

Chapter 10

Assessing Legal and Regulatory Concerns

The legal and legislative issues surrounding PPOs are perhaps some of the most complex of all those associated with PPO development. The purpose of the discussion that follows is to review the principal legal matters applicable to the development and operation of a preferred arrangement.

The major legal concerns facing the PPO are (1) antitrust and other statutory issues, (2) regulation, and (3) liability. More particularly, PPO developers need to know if federal, state, or local statutes act as barriers to the establishment of a preferred arrangement. Paramount among these are federal and state antitrust laws, though others that require consideration include state insurance codes, business and corporate law, health maintenance organization and hospital service corporation acts, and any PPO enabling legislation.[1] PPOs also need to determine whether or not they will be regulated by departments of state government and, if so, in what fashion they will be regulated. Finally, liability issues, contractual and otherwise, that may affect the organizational structuring and eventual operation of the PPO must be carefully researched.

PPO ENABLING LEGISLATION

One authority on legal issues associated with preferred provider organizations remarked recently that as many as 40 states have statutes that preclude or inhibit to some degree the development of preferred provider arrangements. These barriers form a continuum ranging from laws that preclude an insurance company or other entity from interfering in a patient's choice of providers to statutes prohibiting the corporate practice of medicine. In an effort to resolve some of these legal dilemmas, a number of states have enacted preferred provider organization enabling legislation or have modified insurance laws to specifically allow PPO-type arrangements. California, Wisconsin, Virginia, Florida, Colorado, Utah, and Michigan are some of the states in which major legislative action has occurred. In addition, Representative Ron Wyden, an Oregon Democrat, has proposed legislation in the U.S. House of Representatives that should supersede state barriers to the development of preferred provider organizations. It appears, then, that while there may be barriers in some states to the development of PPOs, economic pressure or national legislation may eventually eliminate them.

ANTITRUST IMPLICATIONS FOR PPOs

First, let it be said that some PPO antitrust concerns may, indeed, be legitimate. The preferred provider organization is subject to antitrust scrutiny simply because it is a new form of business venture. Scrutiny of this sort is reasonable and to be expected. But, since a PPO is most often characterized by some combination of providers who were and are competitiors, it may be even more suspect. However, it is necessary to discount both frivolous allegations of antitrust violation that result from the general provider misunderstanding of the concept of a competitive marketplace and those intended to prevent the development of PPOs.

The health care delivery system in general is experiencing increasing antitrust scrutiny. The courts appear unwilling to offer any special treatment to the industry under antitrust and may, in fact, begin to look more often and more closely for antitrust violation. PPOs, then, may expect to receive antitrust attention simply by virtue of the fact that they are a growing part of the health care system, not necessarily because they are unusually suspect.

The "trust" in post-Civil War America was a device utilized by stockholders of competing companies to gain control of several firms through manipulation and to operate them as a monopoly. This particularly pernicious practice was a prime mover in the proposal and enactment of legislation from which public policy toward big business has evolved.

Three major pieces of legislation govern business conduct: the Sherman Antitrust Act of 1890, the Clayton Act, and the Federal Trade Commission Act, both enacted in 1914. All have been amended to reflect new applications made necessary by changes in both the practice of business and the marketplace environment. In general, these statutes are referred to as antitrust laws; however, their flexibility allows for application to other business activity.

The Sherman Antitrust Act provides the basis of most antitrust assessment and litigation. It is broad in scope and flexible enough to deal with a wide variety of antitrust issues. In fact, both the Clayton Act and the Federal Trade Commission Act were written in response to public dissatisfaction with the ambiguity of the Sherman Act. The intent of the Clayton Act was to specify illegal business practices that restrained trade and, thus, to deter behavior that might lead to a monopoly. The Federal Trade Commission Act established a governmental arm empowered to use necessary means to prevent such unfair practice. In contrast, the Sherman Act had dealt with restraint of trade and monopolies on an ex post facto basis.

Section 1 of the Sherman Act addresses all explicit collusion, by those engaged in the same industries, to limit competition among themselves. Interpreted literally, Section 1 would prohibit very nearly all contracts or agreements to conduct business. Historically, however, the courts have interpreted as illegal only those agreements deemed to be unreasonable restraints of trade. Section 2 specifically prohibits both individual or joint maintenance of monopoly power and attempts to monopolize any market.

To be in violation of Section 1 of the Sherman Antitrust Act, business conduct and practice must be judged to be unreasonable in its restraint of trade. The ambiguity of that statutory provision requires that each action to be adjudicated under Section 1 be reviewed and assessed on its own merit. A case decided in this fashion is said to have undergone "rule of reason" analysis. Rule of reason is simply a judicial interpretation that the antitrust statutes prohibit a particular form of business conduct only when it can be shown that such conduct leads to unreasonable consequences. It also prohibits monopoly when such monopoly has been achieved unreasonably.

Certain business practices are deemed so pernicious that the mere existence of them is judged illegal. They are intrinsically evil or at a minimum undesirable. That is to say, no matter the "reasonableness" of the conduct or its intended consequence, the act has been judged by statutory mandate, judicial precedent, or societal consensus to be a priori injurious to a market or individual. These acts are said to be illegal "per se." Merely demonstrating that the conduct occurred is sufficient evidence to elicit a conviction in the courts or an injunction against such activity. The per se rule, then, precludes conduct and/or arrangements that might have been judged reasonable under a comprehensive rule of reason analysis. For this reason, determination of the method of review, being either per se or rule of reason, becomes one of the most critical issues of antitrust proceedings.

Federal antitrust statutes are applicable only to conduct that relates to interstate commerce, thereby protecting the sovereignty of the individual states. The courts, however, have typically given very broad interpretation to the definition of interstate commerce. In fact, recent rulings as to interstate commerce and the health care industry demonstrate this liberal interpretation.

The application of antitrust to health care, and other "professions" as well, has a relatively short history. Prior to 1975, the health care industry enjoyed a long period of virtual immunity from antitrust scrutiny. It had been argued that professional practice was not a form of trade or commerce and antitrust law was, therefore, inapplicable. Exemptions, barriers, and special defenses had shielded professionals from antitrust prosecution and conviction.

After litigation in the lower courts during the '70s, the Supreme Court, in *American Medical Association v. Federal Trade Commission* (1982), upheld the FTC ruling that both the AMA imposition of its guild free-choice ethic and its advertising restrictions on member physicians were illegal.

Several Supreme Court decisions rendered in 1982, in addition to *AMA v. FTC*, carry antitrust significance for the health care industry. Perhaps the most celebrated and cited of these is *Arizona v. Maricopa County Medical Society*. The issue developed when two not-for-profit foundations for medical care, Maricopa Foundation and the Pima Foundation for Medical Care, were created by local medical societies, expressly for the purpose of securing from member physicians agreements to adopt a maximum fee schedule. After agreements were obtained from an overwhelming majority of private physician practitioners in their respective counties, a fee schedule was determined by majority vote of the foundation membership. Commercial carriers of health insurance were then asked to offer health insurance policies based on the adopted maximum fee schedule. Under such a policy, the insured was free to choose any physician, but would receive full reimbursement for care only if the attending physician was a foundation plan member.

The Court ruled, four to three, that agreements among physicians to establish maximum full reimbursement levels for medical care amounted to horizontal price fixing and, as such, were per se violations of federal antitrust statutes. In arguing their case, the defendants asserted that the uniqueness of their plan included a breadth of consumer choice of physician, comprehensive insurance coverage, and a low premium that could not exist without the agreements in question. The Court, however, found that, prior to the inception of the maximum fee schedule, insurers in the geographic area of the plan offered approximately the same breadth of consumer choice and paid about the same number of bills in full.

Furthermore, the Court cited precedents that supported the contention that the agreements among providers were unnecessary to establish maximum fee schedules. Fee schedules had, in fact, been prescribed by purchasers and regulatory agencies. The Court also ruled that the foundations were not legitimate joint ventures by physician members, since the physicians had not entered into "joint arrangements in which persons who would otherwise be competitors pool their capital and share their risks or loss as well as the opportunities for profit." In such cases, those parties are viewed as a single integrated economic entity competing with others in the marketplace and are free from antitrust scrutiny.

Maricopa is viewed as a landmark case because of its ostensible implications for a variety of antitrust violations as they relate to health care delivery. Business practices that are likely to be affected by the *Maricopa* decision are:

- Horizontal price fixing, wherein competing providers set minimum, maximum, or ranges of prices charged to purchasers
- Market divisions, either along geographic or product lines
- Concerted refusals to deal, agreements wherein providers refuse to deal with purchasers of care or alternative delivery systems.

The upshot of these and other court rulings is that the health care industry is no longer subject to special treatment under antitrust scrutiny. The defenses of the past, though some remain viable under special circumstances, are generally invalid. As evolution of a price-competitive health care market continues, the ability of the current antitrust laws to ensure fair competition among actors in the market will become more certain. For the present, however, it appears that existing antitrust statutes, as interpreted by the courts, are flexible enough to eliminate unfair business practice in health care.

Though so much ado has been made of the issue, concerns for PPOs under antitrust scrutiny have been overstated. The basic considerations are the sponsorship of the PPO, the organizational structure of the PPO, and the actual operation of the PPO. The latter two may, in fact, be inextricably intertwined in that the contractual relationships that are the essence of the PPO dictate both structure and operation.

Provider concerns over antitrust matters may, in some situations, serve to inhibit the development of preferred arrangements. Preferred provider organizations intending to structure their programs in a way that may border on violation of antitrust regulations should be prepared to deal with the consequences of their actions. Most PPOs do not seem to wish to risk possible antitrust violation and are structuring themselves accordingly.

In undertaking an assessment of possible antitrust violations, preferred provider organizations and their attorneys should consciously consider the major issues under antitrust scrutiny: (1) the intent of the parties entering into a preferred arrangement and (2) whether or not either the organization or operation of the PPO actually amounts to per se or unreasonable restraint of trade. PPO activity may bring allegations of restraint of trade that fall into three major categories of violation. Those are price fixing, concerted refusals to deal, and tying arrangements.[2] Since these are issues of conduct, the presumption is that the lion's share of questions of antitrust violation might be reviewed under Section 1 of the Sherman Act. This does not, however, preclude analysis under the Clayton Act or by the Federal Trade Commission.

Price Fixing

Horizontal price fixing is characterized by an agreement between or among competitors, either sellers or buyers, the intent of which is to directly or indirectly control market prices. Agreements to conduct a wide variety of activities have been judged per se illegal as horizontal price fixing. Some examples of those are agreements to set minimum prices, maximum fee schedules, uniform price lists, uniform discounting, and concerted price reduction or increase.

Refusals To Deal

Concerted refusals to deal are called, more simply, group boycotts. It is unquestionably permissible for a particular buyer or seller to choose to refrain from dealing with any party. It is not, however, acceptable under antitrust statutes, for buyers or sellers to agree between or among themselves to refrain from dealing with anyone doing business in the marketplace. Such agreements are generally viewed as an attempt to impair the ability of those in the market to operate, or to force a cessation of business in those markets, and are per se violations of both the letter and intent of Section 1 of the Sherman Act.

Tying Arrangements

A tying arrangement exists when a seller requires a buyer agreement to purchase a good or service as a prerequisite to purchasing others. This practice is particularly injurious to marketplace competition when a supplier holds monopoly power over a product through patents or other rights. By requiring a buyer to purchase additional products that seller may extend its monopoly power to those products also, thereby reducing competition further.

Mergers

A lesser consideration is merger. Certain types of mergers are declared to be illegal and may affect PPOs if providers were to merge in order to organize a preferred arrangement. Merger is not in and of itself illegal per se; however, corporations are prevented from merging with or acquiring another firm if such combination will substantially reduce competition. Generally, under the Clayton Act only a probable, rather than actual, reduction of competition need be demonstrated. Thus, this statutory provision is a difficult one to circumscribe, even though the rule of reason is applied.

Horizontal merger involves the combination of firms competing in the same market. A court test determines the extent to which the combination dominates the market. Horizontal mergers may be tolerated if competition is not, in the opinion of the court, significantly impaired. Generally speaking, however, this is the type of merger most often prosecuted under antitrust.

It is often said that the simplest method of avoiding difficulty in most sectors of the legal environment is the application of common sense in our conduct. This axiom holds true in the antitrust environment as well, and it indeed holds true in the case of PPOs. It is clear, then, that common sense organization and operation of the PPO should preclude the vast majority of antitrust concerns.

Sponsorship

Sponsorship is an especially important issue because the activity of the PPO is directed in large part by its controlling interest, i.e., its sponsors. The relationship of sponsorship and operation is crucial in that the question "Who is doing what?" is central to antitrust analysis. Furthermore, certain PPO activity may be perfectly legitimate and pro-competitive for some actors, yet that same activity may be a violation of antitrust law when undertaken by another class of participant. The importance of sponsorship to the PPO arena is further evidenced by the fact that the various models are most often named for sponsors. Third party, purchaser, physician, and hospital-based models are the most prevalent PPO models and are all named for their sponsorship.

Of these, the third party or "broker" model PPO should experience the least antitrust difficulty. These PPOs merely facilitate the provision of service by providers and the purchase of health care by purchasers. That is, they broker, or bring together certain providers and purchasers, and arrange for a mutually beneficial relationship between the parties. There is no controlling interest, either direct or indirect, by any party that buys or sells health care service. Therefore, it would be difficult even to suggest that providers had conspired to fix prices in any way, that purchasers had collectively refused to deal with other providers, or that the participating purchasers and providers had conspired together to deal exclusively with one another.

Since, oftentimes, third-party-sponsored PPOs may negotiate discounts or other special reimbursement arrangements, it may be alleged that they have, in fact, promoted or participated in uniform discounting, maximum or minimum price scheduling, or other per se price-fixing violations. However, if the PPO does not provide or purchase care and is not a legal agent of either provider or purchaser, it should not be judged as having participated in a conspiracy to restrain trade through price fixing. By the same token, the PPO cannot be thought of as having encouraged or facilitated a group boycott. Most contracts that PPOs enter into, with both providers and purchasers, contain a provision that deals specifically with agency. These provisions state very clearly that the contractors are separate entities and that no agency by either party shall exist. Parties considering PPO participation should under no circumstances sign a contract that does not clearly relate that fact. The inclusion of such a provision in a PPO contract is an example of how the application of common sense to the PPO process can begin to alleviate antitrust (and other) concerns.

The Federal Trade Commission, in June 1983, gave its imprimatur to a third-party PPO model developed by Health Care Management Associates, a Moorestown, New Jersey, health care consulting firm. The "Cooperating Provider Program," in the opinion of the FTC, "would not violate the Federal Trade Commission Act or any provision of antitrust law the Commission enforces." The opinion elaborated and allowed that the program as proposed "is likely to be pro-competitive, both by generating competition between . . . providers and by increasing competition among third-party payors." The transmittal cautions that the rendered opinion applied only to the model proposed and that it does not give blanket approval to PPOs of all sorts. However, the FTC stated that it was not implying that all PPOs should mirror the Cooperating Provider Program.[3]

In 1983, the United States Department of Justice issued an advisory opinion seemingly supporting the notion that preferred provider organizations are not at variance with antitrust statutes. The advisory opinion, provided to the Hospital Corporation of America, nicely summarized the Department's view of certain types of preferred provider organizations and antitrust difficulties:

> As a general matter, we believe the emergence of preferred provider organizations can benefit the public by increasing competition among providers and contributing, to some degree, to a decrease in provider's fees. By offering consumers another type of health care delivery system to compete with health maintenance organizations, fee-for-service providers, and other methods of providing medical services, the PPO may spur greater cost-containment efforts and contribute to lower health care costs.[4]

Granted, to date, the majority of such opinions have been rendered vis-à-vis proprietary PPOs. However, the implication is that, no matter the sponsorship, PPOs organized and operated within the bounds of common sense may be encouraged as being pro-competitive.

It is unlikely that purchaser organization of, or participation in, preferred provider organizations will present any more serious antitrust difficulties than should third-party-sponsored ones. Though some employers/purchasers have been reluctant to participate in PPOs because of possible liability, others have expressed concern over antitrust implications, especially members of business health coalitions. The fear seems to be that such activity would be interpreted as a concerted refusal to deal, a group boycott, or other conspiracy to restrain trade.

At a 1983 conference on health care cost containment, Charles D. Weller, a Cleveland attorney and one of the nation's leading authorities on PPO legal issues, interpreted antitrust laws as encouraging purchasers to seek the best possible deal for the delivery of health care services.[5] Furthermore, Walter T. Winslow, Deputy Director of the FTC's Bureau of Competition, has noted, in regard to alternative health care delivery systems, that rivals have attempted to use antitrust statutes to "cripple or even eliminate such alternatives." In a statement before sections of the Minnesota State Bar Association in 1983, Mr. Winslow predicted that "we can surely expect similar efforts for some time to come." However, he followed that prediction with, "But, let me be clear about this, as an antitrust prosecutor I will continue to insist that alternative delivery systems not be formed or operated in ways that injure competition; however, I will also insist that antitrust laws not be misapplied so as to impede alternative arrangements that can bring increased competition through economically desirable integration by health care providers and economically imperative cost containment efforts by third party payors."[6]

These statements offer the purchaser a fresh perspective from which to view the antitrust laws. Traditionally, antitrust statutes have been seen as being preventive, restrictive, and punitive in nature. Most certainly, to the unscrupulous they are and should be. On the other hand, to those who intend to enter the marketplace (be they buyer, seller, or groups of either) and compete freely on the basis of price, quality, service, or value, antitrust laws should be viewed as protective devices that encourage competitive activity. It is this purpose of the antitrust statutes that is most often overlooked.

Marketplace Economics

Purchasers of care are, after all, purchasers of other goods and services. They know that in many cases, greater purchasing power means lower costs. Many enter into joint purchasing agreements with the express intent of using that group buying power to influence the cost of goods and services or to set conditions for their delivery. In fact, competing hospitals, through local associations, often purchase supplies in this fashion. The question becomes "Why should purchasers be unable to apply these same basic principles to the purchase of health care services?" The answer to this question is not "Because inefficient providers, who are unable to compete on the basis of price, may be forced from the market." Rather, there is absolutely no reason why common business practice applied to virtually all other aspects of the marketplace cannot be applied to the purchase of health care. Again, if the intent of purchasers is merely to obtain the best possible price for services and not to impede the ability of any provider to compete on the basis of price, then those purchasers should be at little or no risk of violating antitrust law.

One further extremely important distinction should be made in regard to the antitrust implications of purchaser participation in any PPO, regardless of the model. The success of virtually all PPOs can be traced to the ability of purchasers of care to offer patient/consumer incentives that are sufficiently attractive to cause an alteration of their behavior. There is a vast difference between encouraging and requiring potential patients to use certain providers. Even in exclusive provider arrangements, where no portion of benefits are paid if a patient chooses to use a nonpanel provider, the patient is free to make the choice of provider. It is that freedom of choice that is central to the rebuttal of arguments charging boycott or tying arrangements. Each and every time that a patient requires health care, it is that patient alone who decides whether the provider will be a PPO panel provider or not. If the patient chooses a nonpanel provider and there is an economic disincentive to do so, then the patient must suffer the consequences of irrational economic behavior. The point to be made is that antitrust statutes in no way prohibit a party from encouraging a second party to act in an economically efficient fashion.

In a June 1984 opinion written for a prospective community-sponsored Michigan PPO, William T. Bartlett, a Cincinnati attorney specializing in corporate law, stated that "... the danger of a plan which offers too great an incentive to select limited preferred providers is that it could be found to be a monopoly or to be involved in a 'contract, combination . . . or conspiracy, in restraint of trade. . . .' " Citing specific cases, Bartlett concluded "that substantial encouragement is allowable, and that any scrutiny would be under the 'rule of reason' which looks for anti-competitive purpose or effect."[7] The implication is that PPO participants must exercise prudence in the offering of incentives to potential patients.

The provider-sponsored PPO, from all indications, presents the greatest possibility for antitrust violation. As was discussed, the most serious damage to competition is done by agreements among competitors in a market. The gravest concern derives from the fact that the PPO is comprised of and controlled by providers of care, many of whom may be competitors. While this fact is not true with all provider-sponsored PPO models, it is with most.

Joint Ventures

It is here that the issue of organization is most critical. With proper organization, a provider-sponsored PPO may mitigate antitrust concern. A legitimate joint venture by hospitals, physicians, or a combination of the two may alleviate antitrust problems. Generally, the sponsors will form a separate PPO entity, corporation or otherwise, and share in the ownership of the PPO. The PPO would then function as a negotiator of rates, administrator of contracts, and contractor for administrative services (utilization review, etc.) on behalf of the owner/providers.

Joint ventures are not, however, immune from antitrust litigation. They may, in fact, be subject to scrutiny under either Section 1 of the Sherman Act, or Section 7 of the Clayton Act, which deals with the lessening of competition by tendency to monopolize. The major issue confronting joint venture PPOs is the extent to which they influence the market.[8]

Sponsorship and control of a joint venture model PPO by a large number of providers may be found illegal if it is judged that competition is significantly lessened by such a merger. Recall, however, that mergers are not per se violations of antitrust law. They are analyzed under the rule of reason. For that reason, the intent of the sponsors and the effect of the PPO upon competition are of the utmost importance. If the PPO joint venture is entered into with the intent of providing benefits not previously available, and does so in fact, then it may be deemed lawful, even if competition is lessened. If, however, competition is impeded to a significant degree, an otherwise reasonable arrangement may be found in violation of antitrust statutes.

The FTC has established some guidelines for determining possible antitrust implications for the development of joint arrangements. First, the Commission defines "fully integrated" and "partially integrated" groups. Very simply, a group is fully integrated if members do not compete with one another for patients and partially integrated if the physicians do compete among themselves for patients outside the group. Under these definitions, most provider-sponsored PPOs would be considered partially integrated groups. The FTC states that, in most ordinary cases, a partially integrated group may be composed of up to approximately two-thirds of the physicians in a given market before antitrust concerns may develop. One may draw the concluson that, with proper organization and operation, a PPO may be sponsored by or contract with up to two-thirds of the physician providers located in a single market if the intent of the PPO is to promote competition in the health care marketplace.

Procompetitive Structuring

The issue of integration is strongly related to a sharing of risk. If, in the case of a provider-sponsored PPO, no true economic unit has been created in which there is a reasonable sharing of financial risk by sponsors who naturally compete, agreements among competitors will almost surely be judged to be in violation of antitrust law. In fact, the Maricopa defendants were judged to have fixed prices for this very reason (and others).

Price fixing of this sort is the major area of antitrust concern for PPOs and particularly provider-sponsored PPOs. If participating providers are involved in organizing the PPO, or establishing its fee structure or payment mechanism, the providers may find themselves faced with allegations of price fixing. The extent to which they are involved in those activities influences the risk of antitrust allegation, i.e., the greater the involvement, the greater the risk. A provider-sponsored PPO may avoid price fixing in several ways. It may take the form of a legitimate joint venture or it may arrange for a third party to establish a fee schedule and/or negotiate contracts. Mid-America Health Network located in Kansas City, has arranged for a third party, Voluntary Hospitals of America

(VHA), to establish a schedule of provider reimbursement rates. A provider-sponsored PPO, Mid-America is particularly cognizant of the antitrust issue and followed this course expressly to avoid antitrust problems. Other provider-sponsored PPOs would be well advised to consider this approach when possible.

A number have avoided such difficulty by simply applying thoughtful, procompetitive elements to their structure. These have included the following:

- Fee structures have, simply, not been set.
- Fee structures have been established, but by nonphysician groups. California Foundation for Medical Care, for example, uses nonprovider health care reimbursement panels to establish fee structures.
- Physician participants have agreed to reduce existing (and varying) fee levels by a uniform amount, without specifying minimum or maximum fee levels.
- Set fee structures have been established, but these have resulted from negotiation with purchasers rather than price fixing; this is a subtle but important difference.
- Providers have joined together to function as an integrated economic unit setting prices as a unit. This is provided for and sanctioned by antitrust statutes.
- The provider groups have not dominated the marketplace.

Membership Concerns

Concerted refusals to deal may be charged by providers who are excluded from PPO membership, particularly if they feel that their ability to trade has been damaged. The provider selection process then comes under scrutiny. While developing strident criteria for membership as ensurance of PPO success is strongly recommended, such criteria may or may not carry antitrust implications. The antitrust laws provide that membership in organizations be open to all only if a like organization cannot duplicate the competitive advantages of membership in the first, or that like organizations cannot be formed. It may be presumed that if a provider is excluded from membership in a PPO, that provider may (1) individually compete with the PPO, (2) organize a competing PPO, or (3) join another existing PPO. Since these options are available, excluded providers have difficulty alleging refusal to deal, especially if it can be demonstrated that there was no intent on the part of the PPO to restrain trade. On the other hand, if providers in a single market area combine in a concerted action aimed at preventing the establishment of a PPO, by refusing to participate, they will be guilty of group boycott.

The Bartlett opinion concludes that "the exclusion of certain practitioners from a PPO is acceptable (from the perspective of federal anti-trust law) as long as the exclusion is based upon legitimate business concerns, or upon qualitative peer review and, its effect is not anti-competitive. . . ." It further states that ". . . 'rule of reason' analysis permits any model which is not intended to be anti-competitive or is not anti-competitive in effect."[9]

Exclusive Dealing

Finally, providers and purchasers who enter into PPO agreements may be accused of an exclusive dealing arrangement. This is particularly true if a significant portion of the market is garnered by the PPO. However, the threat of these accusations is small, for good reason. Purchasers participating in PPOs do not make the decision of where their beneficiaries seek care; therefore, the market is, in reality, an open one. The very nature of the PPO precludes an exclusive dealing arrangement.

It is the issue of freedom of choice that truly mitigates antitrust concern. Again, each time that care is necessary, it is the PPO enrollee, the patient/ consumer, who makes the choice as to whether care is sought from a PPO provider or a nonpanel provider. The purchaser who offers a PPO option may attempt to influence that decision by establishing an incentive/disincentive program, but it will not make the choice of who is the provider. As we have noted, the antitrust laws are not intended to prevent the encouragement of economically rational behavior. Furthermore, in most PPOs providers and purchasers will contract with the PPO individually, not as groups. PPOs are merely collections of individual contracts, the nature of which is simply an agreement to act in a certain way if very specific opportunities for the parties to do so are presented to them. That is, providers will sell services and purchasers will pay for service in certain prescribed fashions, should any beneficiaries choose to enter the delivery system under the auspices of PPO enrollment.

It has been said, somewhat facetiously, that anyone can be sued at any time by any other party for any reason. After a nationally recognized attorney involved with PPO development presented an eloquent examination of the multitude of antitrust and liability horrors that awaited PPOs, he was asked whether anyone would have been courageous enough either to have become a homeowner or purchased an automobile had that person discussed the legal responsibilities and liabilities of such ownership with an attorney beforehand. "No way" was the candid answer from the lawyer. Antitrust and other legal concerns are, indeed, valid; they should not, however, artificially and unnecessarily inhibit the development of viable, competitive alternative delivery systems such as the preferred provider organization.

REGULATION AND ITS IMPACT ON DEVELOPING PREFERRED PROVIDER ORGANIZATIONS

A particularly troublesome area for preferred provider organizations is the extent to which the PPO entity is regulated under state laws. An emerging preferred provider organization would obviously want to assess (1) whether it will be regulated under common insurance laws, (2) whether its advertising will be inhibited or reviewed by state bodies, and (3) whether the negotiated payment rates and payment contracts fall under rate review bodies.

Insurance Laws

In general, it appears that preferred provider organizations, at this time, do not fall under insurance codes. However, as preferred provider organizations initiate provider payment systems that border on insurance arrangements, insurance regulations may subsequently result. A preferred provider organization paying a participating primary care physician an annual fee for each subscriber that the physician cares for has a capitated payment arrangement that is governed by insurance codes. An example of one such organization that has adopted the capitation payment for primary care physicians is the Cubic-Scripps Plan for Health, operated by Cubic Corporation in San Diego, California. Primary care physicians in this exclusive provider program are capitated; specialty physicians are paid on a fee-for-service arrangement. When capitation is used, the element of risk is increased, both to the provider and to the patient. The inability of the provider to meet contractual obligations under the capitation arrangement represents a major reason for the inclusion of such arrangements, like health maintenance organizations, under insurance laws. It is reasonable to speculate that when preferred provider or exclusive provider organizations adopt capitation arrangements for participating medical practitioners, the PPO entity will fall under the regulatory powers of state insurance departments.

Preferred provider organizations and exclusive provider arrangements that are evolving toward capitation must, naturally, be prepared to address the additional paperwork, financial reserve requirements, rate hearings, and other public forums that typically accompany insurance regulations. Further, PPOs with these arrangements should have the financial resources to allow them to effectively meet the insurance requirements.

Advertising

In considering the matter of advertising, legal feasibility will determine the extent to which advertising may be undertaken as well as the appropriate scope of advertising. Some states have select prohibitions against the advertising of prices associated with medical services and in states where these exist caution is advised.

Rate Reviews

The variety of hospital rate review programs operating in the United States makes it difficult to outline precisely the way in which a PPO determines whether its activities will be hampered by the rate review process. Those states operating mandatory rate review programs represent the most difficult ones. Preferred provider organizations desiring discounts from participating hospitals may find it impossible to work this out in such states. These states, characterized as "all payor states," mandate not only that hospitals receive approval for the rates they charge insurance companies and other purchasers, but that they also charge each of these purchasers the same amount for comparable services.

PPOs in Maryland, a heavily regulated state, are unable to negotiate hospital discounts. Accordingly, the Greater Baltimore Preferred Provider Organization has emphasized physician practice efficiency as a fundamental organizational principle. Physician practice efficiency, not hospital discounts, has also been a primary marketing tool of the organization.

GENERAL LIABILITY ISSUES

A nebulous, unending continuum of legal issues arises in the area of liability. It can be anticipated that as preferred provider organizations assume greater control and direction over providers of care, through such mechanisms as utilization review and provider selection processes, liability will be a matter of ongoing concern. A few areas of potential liability should be considered in the feasibility stage.

Advertising

The first of these concerns the obligations a PPO may assume as the result of advertised material that leads patients to expect that a certain level of quality medical care and services are available from a competent and highly professional panel of physicians and hospitals. Operational preferred provider organizations, expressly or implicitly warranting the quality of medical care services by virtue of their advertising, should expect to face liability claims in those instances where a PPO patient is able to demonstrate that these obligations were not met. A preferred provider organization may be able to circumvent this area of liability by providing patients and subscribers with explicit disclaimers for the responsibility of meeting qualitative or service standards; such an action, however, would be grossly inconsistent with the marketing strategy of most preferred provider organizations, which is formulated heavily on the ability of the preferred provider organization to provide quality services at a reasonable cost.

Quality of Care

The preferred provider organization's responsibility to provide quality medical services that do not injure patients through neglect or malfeasance is another area of potential liability concern. In particular, developing preferred provider organizations should fully assess two matters influencing the quality of care provided to subscribers/patients. The first is the process by which competent health providers and facilities are selected. By their nature, preferred arrangements may, to some degree, disrupt existing referral patterns between physicians and among hospitals. If legal questions or lawsuits arise from the selection of physicians and hospitals, and if it can be shown that the preferred provider organization seriously interfered with or disrupted medical referral patterns, it is conceivable that liability judgments could be made against PPO entities. That is not to say that this would be the case or that this has been the case. It is important, though, that preferred provider organizations recognize their duty to ensure that the providers selected, and the relationships among those providers, enhance quality medical care and the continuity of that care.

It is possible that variables other than the panel of providers may link a PPO entity to malpractice liability. In the case of *Wickline v. State of California*, a jury awarded $500,000 to the plaintiff, a Medi-Cal recipient, because a utilization review consultant had reduced, from eight to four, the number of additional hospital days requested by the patient's physician. The patient was discharged on the fourth day and developed complications eventually resulting in the amputation of a portion of one leg. In this particular lawsuit, the State of California, which was also the entity responsible for contracting for utilization review, was found negligent.

This decision and others that may have been rendered elsewhere, suggest that PPO entities, particularly those operating aggressive utilization review programs, may be found liable in cases where personal injury results from the negligent application of utilization review standards.

Defamation of Character

Finally, it is important to address the issue of defamation of character. Preferred provider organizations and their agents, e.g., utilization review organizations, make determinations about the appropriateness and necessity for medical care. At times, care may be found to be unnecessary or a particular service, such as an elective hospital admission, may be deemed inappropriate. Patients have a right to an explanation of the reasons for these determinations. In the vigor of applying utilization review standards, however, it may be that an organization could inappropriately link such characteristics as "unnecessary," "inappropriate," and "questionable," with the care rendered by a particular physician. Depending on the circumstances of a particular case, the irresponsible communication of such to patients and/or the conscious defamation of a physician's character by such communication may serve as grounds for defamation litigation.

Dealing with Constraints

There are, no doubt, numerous other liability issues to be considered. These represent merely some of the more prominent. The potential liability and legal ramifications associated with preferred provider organization development often appear to be unending. Very likely, many a potential PPO participant or developer has shied away from PPO association because of such concerns. But liability issues face all persons at virtually all times. However, when reasonable, rational action is undertaken by sincere, competent individuals and institutions, the probability of liability should be minimal. Yes, it should always be considered, but it should not be overstated.

NOTES

1. "Health Law Outlook," Wood, Lucksinger & Epstein, Vol. 2, No. 7, June, 1983, p. 4.

2. H. Robert Halper, "Law Notes," *Business and Health* (Washington Business Group on Health) 1, no. 3 (January/February 1984): 48.

3. Advisory Opinion, Office of the Secretary, Federal Trade Commission, Washington, D.C. in Response to a Request From Health Care Management Associates, Moorestown, N.J., June 7, 1983.

4. Advisory Opinion issued by William F. Baxter, Office of the Assistant Attorney General, U.S. Department of Justice, Antitrust Division. In response to a request by Hospital Corporation of America, September 21, 1983.

5. Charles D. Weller, "A Lawyer's View of PPOs and the Antitrust Issue." Presentation at the National Conference on Health Care Cost Containment sponsored by the National Association of Employers on Health Care Alternatives, Chicago, Illinois, October 13, 1983.

6. Walter T. Winslow, "Antitrust and Alternative Health Care Systems," Statement before the Antitrust and Health Care Sections of the Minnesota State Bar Association, May 25, 1983.

7. William T. Bartlett, Advisory Opinion from *Preferred Provider Organizations and Grand Haven, Michigan: A Feasibility Assessment* (Cincinnati, Oh.: Morgan Bigae Institute, June 1984).

8. R.E. Strombert, M.S. Duncheon, and J.S. Goldman, "PPOs and the Antitrust Laws," *Hospitals* (October 16, 1983): 67.

9. op cit., Bartlett.

Part IV

The Future

Chapter 11

The Evolution and Outcome of Preferred Provider Arrangements

The evolution of PPOs is occurring so rapidly that speculation about the future of the movement is risky and clearly a subjective enterprise. Yet, even with this observation, certain trends seem to be taking place and, as they do, those watching this phenomenon are compelled to gaze momentarily into health care's crystal ball.

The future holds some interesting as well as distressing changes for PPOs and their participants. In the short term, physicians can be expected to compete with hospitals for the increasing fixed level of resources channeled into the health care system. Future-oriented hospitals, however, will recognize that joint ventures with physicians can be structured to symbiotically enhance competitiveness with other entities. These PPO joint ventures will involve substantial risk assumption, an ingredient largely lacking in current joint ventures.

The distinction between PPOs and HMOs will diminish and, in the long run, provide the springboard to health care's next evolutionary phase: The Comprehensive Health Care Delivery System.

Quality of care will be improved throughout this evolution, not because of altruism but for patently economic and competitive purposes. PPOs and price sensitivity will result in the same kind of marketplace changes that occur in any other competitive environment; weak and inappropriately priced competitors will lose business, go bankrupt, and eventually dissolve. In health care this refers specifically to hospitals.

The possibility of large-scale hospital closures can be inhibited only by the very nemesis of the PPO movement: regulation. The scenario summarized above will hinge on the manner in which national and state policy makers confront this challenge of hospital insolvency.

Oddly, the future and evolution of the PPO movement seems to be heading on a collision course with the past. Alternative delivery systems have grown and attracted major purchaser attention because of the inadequacies and failures of regulation. The serious problems surfacing from PPO growth and that of other alternative systems ironically seem to require regulatory-based solutions largely inconsistent with price sensitivity and competition. These trends are examined more closely below.

HOSPITAL-PHYSICIAN COMPETITION

There can be no doubt that the fragile nature of hospital-physician relationships will be increasingly strained by the myriad of health care changes taking place. On one hand, it is absolutely essential for hospitals to nurture cooperative bonds with their physicians. The expansion of payment systems that put hospitals at financial risk for the cost of care generated by their medical staffs mandates a level of cost efficiency and cooperation unparalleled in medical care. PPOs are serving as one of the most important channels for the expansion of payment systems that place serious direct economic pressure on hospitals to control medical costs.

While hospitals desperately need the cooperation and commitment of physicians, the reverse is far less true. Emerging trends in employee benefits, physician reimbursement policies, and physician incentive arrangements are offering doctors new financial incentives to use hospital facilities as the setting of last resort. Employees are being given incentives (or disincentives) to acquire outpatient care, much of which is delivered in physician office complexes. PPO payment approaches are being structured so that physicians are paid decreasing fees for minor surgical procedures performed, respectively, at the office, on an outpatient basis in a hospital, and on an inpatient basis. Incentive systems, like that established through Blue Cross/Blue Shield of Virginia, are formulated on similar physician practice behavior.

The financial resources of the health care system are becoming increasingly fixed. The unlimited reservoir of the past is gone. In this environment, physicians will aggressively compete with hospitals for economic resources.

This scenario portrays a particularly pessimistic future for hospitals and their relationship with physicians. But this need not be the case for visionary, creative hospitals. Such facilities are already recognizing that they have the ability to construct innovative hospital-physician ventures which, in themselves, reward quality, efficient behavior. This in turn, provides the competitive edge that will allow some facilities to capture the commitment and loyalty of physicians in an environment filled with wedges of division.

SYMBIOTIC JOINT VENTURES

The second systemwide trend, then, is seen in those symbiotic physician-hospital joint ventures which are the tool that can minimize or eliminate the economic competition between a medical staff and its respective hospital. The PPO has been and will continue to be a major type of symbiotic joint venture.

A symbiotic joint venture implies that all participating parties reap the benefits of mutual interaction. This is a critical point because the mere formation of a joint program, such as a hospital-physician PPO, may not necessarily be symbiotic. Concisely, successful hospital-physician joint ventures are and will be those embodying four characteristics. The venture will assume financial risk; it will limit the risk by involving only high-quality, efficient providers; participants will have an economic commitment to the venture; and, provider participants will reap financial rewards commensurate with their individual performance and that of the joint venture.

In practical terms, this means the following. First, the acceptance of financial risk opens financial opportunities. Purchasers like Medicare, Arizona's AHCCCS (Arizona Health Care Cost Containment System), San Diego's Medically Indigent Adult (MIA) program, and a variety of state medical programs are increasingly offering provider groupings fixed-sum contracts to provide care for defined populations. Provider groupings like joint venture PPOs are, accordingly, given the opportunity to generate attractive profits if care is judiciously and economically delivered. Fixed-sum contracts and provider bidding represent a trend of significant proportion.

Second, the assumption of risk means that joint venture PPOs will no longer be able, or willing, to absorb financial losses resulting from uncommitted, inefficient providers. Efficiency credentialing, a trend itself, represents a mechanism for resolving this problem. The efficiency credentialing might be based on nonacute profiles or collected utilization data. Regardless of the source, PPOs and affiliated providers can be expected to develop and rigidly apply a credentialing process based on quantitative standards that restricts participation by those with casual practice patterns.

Third, joint venture PPOs have and will continue to require a financial commitment to the venture. Financial participation produces an environment in which all involved have a common economic interest: to survive and thrive in a competitive marketplace by delivering cost-efficient, quality medical care. In this respect, joint venture PPOs can be expected to gravitate toward stock ownership by the physicians and hospital(s) involved. It is easy to imagine that the price of such stock (i.e., PPO participation) and the annual financial rewards to its owners (dividends resulting from efficient performance) will advance rapidly for those ventures that establish successful market positions. The establishment of an equity environment, increases in that equity because of marketplace achievements, and the generation of profit through the successful assumption of risk, together, represent the fourth characteristic of successful physician-hospital joint ventures of the future.

The PPO movement and, more generally, the emergence of price sensitivity, will serve to bring the most visionary physicians and hospitals together as quasi-economic units. The economic units may at first begin as joint venture PPOs. They will move incrementally toward the organizational state of the Comprehensive Health Care Delivery System (CHCDS). They will be economic alliances composed of frequently autonomous, yet contractually linked, providers: physicians, hospitals, nursing homes, pharmacies, home health agencies, etc. It will be in the direct economic interest of providers to affiliate only with others capable of meeting the stringent quality and efficiency demands of the health marketplace.

COMPREHENSIVE HEALTH CARE DELIVERY SYSTEMS

The evolution of PPOs to CHCDSs represents a third systemwide, major trend. Group practice, staff and IPA types of HMOs, through the addition of PPO-like and other products, are also broadening the ways in which they deliver care. The evolution of comprehensive health care delivery systems means, ironically, the end to health maintenance organizations and preferred provider organizations. In the health system of the future, prepaid and preferred provider products will be offered simultaneously by the new CHCDSs. Organizations that fail to evolve into diversified CHCDSs will limit market success and, ultimately, organizational viability.

LIMITING CONSUMER CHOICE OF PROVIDERS

The predicted evolution of PPOs, and other groupings, into CHCDSs is being stimulated by a fourth system trend, which is philosophical in nature. There is a growing recognition that purchasers and those they buy care for must make certain compromises to restrain medical inflation. They can either allow unlimited choice of providers, facing cutbacks in benefit levels and indirectly the quality of care that can be purchased with available resources, or restrict access to only cost-efficient providers, thereby allowing comprehensive benefit levels. The growth of HMOs and reported preferred panel use rates imply that consumers would rather limit choice than the benefits. This apparent philosophical trend, in combination with the growth of employee cost sharing expected for the remainder of this decade, suggests that market forces will clearly favor comprehensive health care delivery systems.

PPOs AND THE ENHANCEMENT OF QUALITY

The quality of care delivered by PPOs, and their CHCDS successors, is likely to be debated in a most spirited fashion for some time. There is reason to believe that, contrary to the view of many skeptics, serious and successful PPOs will advance rather than retard the quality of medical care.

PPOs ·competing for business in any given community may initially exhibit observable differences in their cost-containment performance. Over time, though, price competition will have two effects: (1) costly PPOs will lose business and (2) those that remain will eventually parallel each other in costs and cost efficiency. Purchasers want both cost efficiency and quality, and it is the latter item that will be consistently monitored, evaluated, and improved upon as a market strategy for distinguishing one PPO from others. Ironically, quality will be positively manipulated for distinctly economic purposes. Physician selection and monitoring will reflect this reality. PPOs will be unwilling to tolerate inefficient or qualitatively deviant providers because the financial well-being of the organization will be at stake.

Classic examples of quality enhancement resulting from economic imperatives can be found in the auto industry of the 1980s. At Ford, "quality is job one." Chrysler puts its "risk" where its mouth is; it will guarantee an engine for five years or 50,000 miles. The extensive market penetration of the U.S. auto industry by high-quality, long-lasting Japanese imports forced American automakers to place a new, serious emphasis on quality. The same phenomenon appears to be an immediate outgrowth of the PPO movement. Those who fail to see this trend underestimate the growing sophistication and aggressiveness of purchasers.

HOSPITAL INSOLVENCIES

The evolution of preferred panel arrangements will be accompanied by other tangents. Not all of these will be pleasant. Perhaps one of the most disturbing influences of PPO evolution (and price sensitivity in general) will be experienced by a select group of acute care institutions: (1) heavily indebted hospitals, (2) teaching and research facilities, and (3) institutions serving the indigent. For a variety of reasons these hospitals will find it difficult, if not impossible, to maintain long-term linkages with preferred panel or other alternative delivery arrangements.

Facilities that have embarked on major capital programs and, in the process, assumed relatively large levels of indebtedness represent a serious concern. Unless such institutions are gifted with unprecedented efficiency, overflowing philanthropy, or truly unique market advantages (e.g., an established, undisputed reputation), they will find that vast debt levels inhibit PPOs from associating with them or, equally probable, such institutions will be forced to extend sizable discounts to PPOs. Discounting makes short-term sense if lost revenue can be regained through volume increases. In the long term, though, discounting becomes an avenue to further financial difficulty unless tangible efficiency gains occur.

The decade of the '80s will not be kind to excessively indebted hospitals. Communities in which price sensitivity and alternative delivery systems have grown rapidly will see hospital bankruptcies. The continued phase-in of DRG-based payment, the inclusion of capital costs in these payments, the growth of PPOs and other alternative delivery systems, and at-risk hospital reimbursement approaches will culminate, in the post-1986 era, to bring about these bankruptcies. The principal locations and extent of bankruptcies is not easy to assess. What can be said, though, is that these bankruptcies will measurably affect the tax-exempt hospital bond market, crushing investor confidence in this investment avenue. Bankruptcies will make it difficult and extremely costly for community hospitals nationally to tap the historically generous, low-cost tax-exempt market for needed capital improvements in the latter years of this decade.

Teaching and research centers will also face problems in the establishment of favorable PPO relationships. The high cost of teaching and research will discourage serious PPOs from maintaining such relationships or, on the other hand, will encourage them to tenaciously negotiate large discounts. In either event, the competitive ability of teaching and research centers will be negatively influenced by nonpatient care costliness. Facilities serving the indigent will, likewise, be of limited appeal to PPOs. The primary market of PPOs are employed groups; candidly, facilities with large indigent patient bases have not and will not be viewed as marketing assets.

THE FUTURE MEETS THE PAST

The pessimistic future facing teaching and research centers, facilities caring for sizable indigent populations, and the probable truncation of the tax-exempt hospital bond market are each matters of serious national concern. These problems are not the direct result of the PPO movement, but the PPO explosion with its emphasis on cost efficiency and control is contributing substantially to them. There is no doubt that they require immediate attention; however, the alternatives for their resolution are limited. Bankruptcies can be avoided and the financial needs of teaching and indigent-oriented facilities met by two fundamental approaches—subsidy and/or rate regulation. Subsidies for faltering institutions could be provided, but by whom and at what cost? "All-payor" rate regulation would mandate parity among payors and ensure that the minimal financial needs of institutions are equitably met by all who purchase services. But price competitiveness and the PPO movement could be substantially retarded, if not eliminated, by "all-payor" rate regulation.

Paradoxically, the very survival of the PPO movement may hinge on a conscious effort not to achieve its full competitive potential, for doing so will, in the short term, stimulate hospital financial problems that society may be unwilling to allow. Regardless, the ultimate outcome can only be that the PPO movement will greatly change the face of America's contemporary medical care system. It is a challenging and interesting time.

Index

H

G

Q

Quality of care, 27
  future outlook for, 187, 190-191
  as potential liability issue, 181-182

R

Rapid claims payment, 28
Rate review programs, 180-181
Rate structure alternatives, 154-157
Reagan administration, and health
  planning system, 10
Refusals to deal, 172
Regulation, 179-180, 187-188
  advertising, 180
  insurance laws, 180
  rate review, 180-181
Regulation issues, 167
Relationship between hospitals and
  medical staffs, 28-29
Relative value scale (RVS), 21,
  89
Religious affiliation of facilities, and
  population mix assessment, 143
Reputation of facilities, and
  participation assessment, 143-144
Request for proposal (RFP), 93-95
Retrospective review, 107-108
Revenue impact analysis for hospitals,
  153-154
Revenue sources, 145, 147-148
  identification, 150-152
Revenues, and cost of operation,
  145
RFP. See Request for proposal
Risk sharing, 26
  encouragement of, 96
  and payment per admission, 93
Risk-sharing payment mechanisms,
  43
Robert Wood Johnson Foundation, 23,
  95
Rohr Industries, 26

S

San Diego Committee for Affordable
  Health Care, 95
San Diego Employers Health Cost
  Coalition, 105, 108
San Diego Foundation for Medical
  Care, 94
San Diego PPO, Inc., 21, 22, 94-95
San Diego Program for Affordable
  Health Care, 23
ScrippsCare, 146
The Scripps Clinic, 41, 42
Scripps Memorial Hospital Healthcare
  Management System, 148
Second opinion programs, 105-106
Self-funded employers, 119, 120
Self-funding, cost savings resulting
  from, 131
Self-funding of employee health
  benefits, 35-36, 41
  growth of, 8-9
Semifixed costs, 153, 154, 164
Semivariable costs, 153, 154, 164
Service area delineation, 122-123
Services selection, and consumer
  incentives to alter, 66-67
Sherman Antitrust Act of 1890,
  168-169, 171, 176
Specialty participation assessment,
  142
Sponsorship of preferred provider
  organizations, 37-39, 173-175
Stability of preferred provider
  organizations, 121
Stoner and Associates, 107
Subscriber needs, 121-122
Supreme Court decisions, and health
  care industry, 170-171
Symbiotic joint ventures, 188-190

T

Third-party-sponsored preferred
  provider organizations, 173, 174

About the Authors

S. Brian Barger has more than a decade of experience in health care and cost containment. He has written, spoken, and consulted widely on medical care cost containment in his present capacity as President and Chief Executive Officer of the Morgan Bigae Institute, which has provided cost containment assistance to Fortune 50 companies, business health coalitions, hospital trustee groups, chambers of commerce, third party administrators, universities, health planning agencies, hospitals, and physicians.

His ideas on cost containment have been presented before national and state legislative bodies and, in 1979, he was an invitee to, and participant in, The White House Briefing on Hospital Cost Containment convened by President Jimmy Carter. In addition to his past election to the Governing Council of The American Public Health Association, Mr. Barger's leadership in the health field has been recognized by his inclusion in International Men of Achievement (8th edition, 1981) and Community Leaders of America (12th edition, 1982).

David G. Hillman is Senior Vice President and cofounder of the Morgan Bigae Institute. He has held various executive and technical positions during the past fifteen years, including service as Director of Data Management for a midwestern health planning agency and as owner of Geo-graphics, a computer graphics design firm. His experience also includes five years as a U.S. Naval air traffic controller. In addition, he has served as President and Treasurer of Dencare, Inc., a Cincinnati-based dental PPO of which he was a major developer.

Mr. Hillman has lectured in Geography at the University of Cincinnati and travelled Europe extensively while residing for two and one-half years in Iceland. His professional accomplishments were acknowledged by his inclusion in the 1982 edition of Outstanding Young Men of America.

H. Randall Garland has twenty-two years of experience in health care. He presently serves as Executive Vice President and consultant on health economics and financing to CORVA, the Cincinnati area health planning agency. Prior to coming to CORVA in 1969, Mr. Garland spent nine years at Blue Cross of Southwest Ohio, with various professional responsibilities in corporate research and underwriting, claims processing, analysis of medical care utilization, and the development of health care cost trends and economic forecasting.

He lectures at the University of Cincinnati and Xavier University in his capacity as adjunct professor. He has been an advisor to a wide spectrum of organizations including the Ohio Department of Public Welfare (Medicaid), the Bureau of Health Planning in the U.S. Department of Health and Human Services, the National Center for Health Services Research, and the Ohio Department of Health.

During 1983–84, Mr. Garland served as an appointed member of the Ohio Governor's Commission on Ohio Health Care Costs.